D1416880

By the same authors

The Chinese Way to Healing:
Many Paths to Wholeness

The HIV
Wellness
Sourcebook

The HIV Wellness Sourcebook

Misha Ruth Cohen,
O.M.D., L.Ac.

WITH KALIA DONER

*An
East/West
Guide to
Living Well
with HIV/AIDS
and Related
Conditions*

AN OWL BOOK

HENRY HOLT AND COMPANY

NEW YORK

Henry Holt and Company, Inc.
Publishers since 1866
115 West 18th Street
New York, New York 10011

Henry Holt® is a registered
trademark of Henry Holt and Company, Inc.

Published in Canada by Fitzhenry & Whiteside Ltd.,
195 Allstate Parkway, Markham, Ontario L3R 4T8.

Library of Congress Cataloging-in-Publication Data
Cohen, Misha Ruth.
The HIV wellness sourcebook: an East/West guide to
living well with HIV/AIDS and related conditions /
Misha Ruth Cohen, with Kalia Doner.
p.   cm.
Includes index.
ISBN 0-8050-5117-1 (alk. paper)
1. AIDS (Disease)—Complications—Alternative treatment.
2. AIDS (Disease)—Complications—Treatment.   3. Medicine, Chinese.
I. Doner, Kalia.   II. Title.
RC607.A26C639   1998   97-31830
616.97′92061—dc21   CIP

Henry Holt books are available for special promotions
and premiums. For details contact: Director, Special Markets.

First Edition 1998

Technical illustrations by Nadine Lurie of Vital Presentations
Acupuncture illustrations by Robin Michals

Printed in the United States of America
All first editions are printed on acid-free paper. ∞

10   9   8   7   6   5   4   3   2   1

Stanton, Amanda, Louis, Susan,

Julius, Gary, Tim, Keith, Mark,

Joseph, Steven, Hap, Mandy, Clorice,

David, Sandy, Joe, Margaret . . .

We all have a list that we carry in our heads—

the list of those we've lost, but who inspire us

every day to move forward, to keep heart,

to never waver from pursuit of a cure.

Acknowledgments

I would like to thank many people for their tireless support, reading and editing this manuscript, talking for many hours in person and on the phone, and standing by me when exhaustion made it difficult to say or write one more word.

Thanks to my coauthor Kalia Doner, whose ability to take my thoughts and words and turn them into a truly readable form always amazes me. Thanks also to my agent Regula Noetzli, whose interest and help keeps the process going. To David Sobel, our editor, whose keen insight increased the readability of this book, and to his associate Amy Rosenthal; to Nadine Lurie, whose technical illustrations help make complex ideas understandable, and Robin Michals for her wonderful drawings of the acupuncture channels and points; to my personal assistant Molly Hall, who has helped me keep deadlines and acted as liaison; to Gary Smith and the staff at Chicken Soup Chinese Medicine, who kept the clinic running smoothly; to all the practitioners who have taught me, whom I have taught, and with whom I have shared insights, frustrations, and accomplishments.

And especially thanks to my wonderful friends, colleagues, comrades, clients, and intimates, Donald Abrams, Barbara Adler, Beth Custer, Donna Futterman, Kelly Hill, Naomi Jay, Dorothy Kleffner, Lark Lands, Mary Romeyn, Abelardo Rosas, Carla Wilson, and Katharine Woodruff, whose knowledge and guidance so enriched the book.

And above all, to the women and men with HIV/AIDS whom I have met or never met, known slightly or deeply, cried with, and healed with over the last fifteen years—you truly inspire me and keep my spirit strong every day. Thank you.

Contents

Chinese medicine has given me great gifts that help imbue my mind with a peaceful clarity: Those gifts are the ability to see life as a unity of opposites; to accept the fact that struggle and reward are joined; and to take consolation in the certainty that sickness and healing can exist at the same time in the same person. It is these revelations that have shaped my belief in the wholeness of existence and continue to guide my approach to working with people with HIV.

People with AIDS have given me great gifts that imbue my spirit with an all-encompassing feeling of respect and awe. Over and over I am struck by the resilience and determination that you possess. I am honored to be allowed to share in your process of coping with the consequences of this difficult disease. And I want to express my thanks to those of you who are living with HIV for allowing me to come into your life, gain wisdom from your struggle, and participate in your healing process.

I hope you'll join with me now on a journey exploring the paths to wholeness that are available when Western medical treatments and Chinese medicine therapies are used together to help those of you with HIV/AIDS manage your medical care and take charge of your self-care.

I am convinced that people with HIV infection can create the most effective treatment program by combining Chinese and Western medicine under the umbrella of the Chinese philosophy of healing. This provides the best chance for prolonged survival and minimal complications. That's why, no matter what symptoms a person has, when someone comes to me for treatment I help them create a comprehensive program to restore balance to the mind/body/spirit as a whole. In addition, when called for, I also focus on providing symptomatic relief.

Sometimes that means suggesting Western and other therapies in addition to Chinese medicine. I believe strongly in doing anything you can to help an individual create wholeness and wellness in his or her life.

For example, when someone comes to the clinic with diarrhea, we run a

Western stool test at a special laboratory, Great Smokies, to see if the diarrhea is being caused by organisms that can be treated by antibiotics, herbal formulas, and/or nutritional supplements. When I receive the results, I consult with the person's Western doctor to determine whether antibiotics are the best solution, or whether we can proceed with herbal formulas and nutritional supplements alone. Often we design a protocol using all three treatments.

At the same time, I use Chinese medicine to restore balance to the mind/body/spirit and when necessary to help alleviate potentially toxic side effects of the Western medicine. I've observed that when Western drug therapy causes anemia, Chinese blood tonics and vitalizers often help reverse the reaction.

In some circumstances we may not use Western therapy at all. Chronic sinusitis is especially suited to a combination of acupuncture and herbal medicine. And neuropathy can be treated quite well using acupuncture, moxibustion, massage, and in some cases herbs.

Choosing the most appropriate therapy or combination of therapies to restore harmony to the whole mind/body/spirit gives the person with HIV/AIDS an opportunity to put together a powerful regimen of healing.

—*Misha Ruth Cohen*

Introduction

BY JAMES W. DILLEY, M.D.

The AIDS epidemic presents society and individuals with multiple challenges. As a psychiatrist devoted to reducing the impact of the epidemic, my work for the past sixteen years has been focused on helping those who are HIV-positive improve their quality of life and on bringing a mental health perspective to preventing the spread of HIV.

Today, advances in treatment have changed the way the medical community approaches HIV disease, and people living with HIV are finding that they are staying healthier longer. Yet, significant challenges remain. Not the least of these are managing the psychological stress that accompanies the diagnosis of a life-threatening disease and the emotional difficulties associated with adhering to a complex regimen of antiretroviral drug therapy. Depression and anxiety continue to be frequent companions of the disease and mental health interventions continue to be a critical component of AIDS care. Those who are HIV-positive can best combat these difficulties by learning to take control of their life, learning to become a partner with health care providers, and actively participating in decisions about their care. This book helps them do just that.

The integration of Chinese and Western medicine laid out in *The HIV Wellness Sourcebook* provides those who are HIV-positive with an opportunity to focus on "healing" in the largest sense. It allows them the chance to learn about their disease and to take active steps to allay some of the symptoms associated with HIV and related disorders.

In addition, the therapeutic programs in *The HIV Wellness Sourcebook* combine self-care with integrated medical care and by their very nature help quell some of the anxiety that living with HIV inevitably generates. These programs emphasize the role of the mind and spirit in the health of the body, clearly explaining the Chinese medicine method of integrating the three components of human existence. They promote an understanding of the importance of being connected to others and of cultivating a social support network—which have repeatedly been shown to be important to successfully managing HIV.

Studies have shown that chronically ill people who take an active approach to their health care are much more likely to enjoy a better quality of life, and in some instances better physical health, than those who do not. I believe that one of the most powerful ways to improve the quality of life of those who are HIV-positive is to offer them as many tools as possible in their search for what works best for them. One significant tool is provided by the wisdom and insights of Eastern healing arts.

JWD
Founder and Executive Director,
University of California San Francisco AIDS Health Project
since 1984 and Clinical Professor of Psychiatry

The HIV
Wellness
Sourcebook

PART I

A View
from the East:

Toward Understanding
Chinese Medicine and Its Ability
to Improve the Treatment
of People with HIV Infection

The wise person never tries to see into
the heart of a mystery with one eye closed
—*Anonymous proverb*

1

In Honor of Those
Living with HIV/AIDS

When I think of all the friends I've lost to this damned disease, I try
not to be bitter or depressed—and that's hard. But I believe their lives
had meaning and glory, no matter how short. And their thwarted
desire to live fires me up with an almost ferocious desire to beat this
thing. That's why I believe we each must put ourselves to work to
find the best treatments available from all medical traditions and push
for unflinching public support in pursuit of a cure.

—Gregory, 42, artist, diagnosed in 1986

No fancy talk. No long, drawn-out explanations. Time is best spent in
the practice of healing and self-healing, not talking about it. I want you to
jump into this book and become familiar with the general Chinese medicine
practices and targeted programs that are suited to your specific needs at this
time. (You can revisit the various chapters over and over, as your needs
change.) For the wonder of Chinese medicine—particularly when used as the
philosophical underpinning for healing—is that it offers immediate and deeply
moving opportunities to change how you feel today, this hour, now.

WHAT THIS BOOK OFFERS YOU

The HIV Wellness Sourcebook takes you through a concise course in Chinese
medicine practices, offering a fresh perspective on how best to prevent and
treat the disharmonies associated with HIV infection. You'll learn how to
maintain strength using Chinese dietary therapy, Qi Gong exercise and meditation, acupuncture and moxibustion, herbal therapy, and other natural therapies. These taken together provide a comprehensive treatment program for
all people with HIV/AIDS.

This book reveals how Western and Eastern medicine's views of the syndrome complement each other. And you'll find out how to blend Chinese and
Western medical therapies.

In addition to the comprehensive treatment program, in Part IV *The HIV
Wellness Sourcebook* outlines more programs, such as managing digestive

disorders or handling addiction in the presence of HIV infection, that will help you guide your Chinese (and Western) practitioner and shape your self-care. You'll expand your understanding of how to best heal your mind/body/spirit.

FINDING THE PATH

The journey I took to bring Chinese medicine to bear on the challenge of dealing with HIV infection started with my unyielding commitment to making optimal medical care available to all people. When the AIDS epidemic began, my clinic, Quan Yin Acupuncture and Herb Center, was the first in San Francisco to openly welcome people with HIV infection and offer them high-quality, affordable, full-service Chinese medicine therapies. In 1984, Western medicine could offer only rudimentary treatments for some opportunistic infections, and many long-term survivors were using acupuncture, herbs, and other natural therapies.

Later, when the pharmaceutical companies began offering antiviral drug therapies, people with HIV infection continued to use our services because the treatments worked. Over the years, as our skill developed, we were able consistently to relieve symptoms, eradicate some problems completely, and increase quality of life.

Now, 15 years later, there are Western treatments for many opportunistic infections. Early intervention and careful screening have increased longevity. Triple-drug cocktails with protease inhibitors reduce viral load counts to undetectable levels for some people. But Chinese medicine continues to have a vital role to play:

- Modern Chinese herbal formulas now exist to ease specific HIV-related disharmonies. (For detailed information see Chapter 7, on herbal therapy, and Appendixes 2 and 3.)
- There are many HIV-associated infections that Western medicine cannot adequately remedy, but that traditional Chinese medicine can treat very effectively.
- Chinese medicine can ease adverse reactions to Western drug therapies, allowing for continued use of those drugs—an important partnership when the medication is being taken to prevent devastating opportunistic infections.
- Chinese medicine offers an integrated approach to healing, and that, I believe, is essential if the quest for wellness is to be effective. On the other hand, Western medicine does not address health problems that are associated with disharmonies in the underlying constitution of an individual; it does not usually extend treatment to remedy the subtle but far-reaching domino effect that HIV infection can have on all the organ systems; and it does not often offer treatments for a troubled spirit. The

Chinese medicine practitioner's essential task, when working with someone with HIV infection, after learning all the facts, is to help keep the
spirit steady and safe while applying strong treatment to the body.

CHALLENGES FACING THE COLLABORATION OF EAST AND WEST

Despite—or perhaps because of—the differences between Chinese and Western therapies, their practitioners are able to work side by side in clinical set-
tings. Day to day their effectiveness together is apparent to practitioners and
to people with HIV. But when it comes to "proving" what is observed clini-
cally, they conflict with each other: The methodology of Western research
isn't well suited to studying the effectiveness of Chinese medicine therapies
because Chinese medicine treats each person as an individual. (In Western
controlled studies all participants are assumed to be basically identical.)

Clearly, controlled studies are needed to evaluate the impact of Chinese
medicine, but until now such investigations have not allowed for the com-
plexities of how Chinese medicine works. New research methodology is
needed, and current attempts in that direction will take a few years to evolve.

It's my goal to be a catalyst in that process and I'm thrilled that along with
San Francisco's Community Consortium and principal investigator Donald
Abrams, M.D., I am involved in a study of Health Concern's Marrow Plus herb
formula. The study, funded by Bastyr University in Seattle from a grant from
the National Institutes of Health's Office of Alternative Medicine, has a sub-
group of participants who receive a Chinese medicine diagnosis. We try to
predict who will respond to the herbal formula and then evaluate the results.
The study is slated to be completed in 1998.

Such joint efforts improve communication between Western and traditional Chinese practitioners enormously. Those who practice Chinese medicine are learning to understand and incorporate principles learned from
Western research and treatment concepts. And Western-trained doctors are
researching Eastern methods of treatment[1] and are referring their clients to us
for therapy. To track the evolution of Chinese medicine's application to HIV/
AIDS and the growing collaboration between Western and Chinese medicine
in the treatment of the syndrome, see the time line in Appendix 1.

2

The Powers of Chinese Medicine: Understanding the Basics

I attribute a lot of my emotional well-being to Chinese medicine. It makes me feel more grounded—more like myself. I also like the way the relationship with a Chinese medicine doctor makes healing a cooperative affair. And the treatments have reduced a lot of negative side effects from the pharmaceuticals I'm taking. All in all, there are just a lot of benefits that you might not expect.

—Stanley, 33, businessman, diagnosed in 1995

To use Chinese medicine you don't have to understand its underlying philosophy or principles. You can take the herbs, receive acupuncture, and try other therapies much as you would take a pill—Western style—and you will still reap considerable benefits.

But a curious thing happens when you use Chinese medicine: Its transforming power insinuates itself into your unconscious as the treatments strengthen your mind/body/spirit. You find, despite your lack of understanding of how it works or what it can do, that repeated exposure to the basic treatments—herbs, acupuncture, dietary therapy, Qi Gong exercise, and meditation—changes you in subtle but far-reaching ways. You become more tuned in to your physical and spiritual self. You become aware of the profound impact of your breath on your physical and mental well-being; you begin to sense the flow of Qi, the life force, through your body; you tune in to your own mental and physical strengths and imbalances; you learn to rejoice in the interconnectedness of all life experience.

This transformation creates a sense of empowerment that's particularly important in dealing with a chronic disorder such as HIV disease, which can erode your sense of control over your own body and make you feel estranged from your physical and spiritual self.

Putting yourself within the Eastern frame of mind will help you maximize the effectiveness of Western treatments (and lessen the negative side effects). You'll also be better able to manage HIV-associated disorders and diseases, such as sinusitis and chronic diarrhea, which often resist Western treatments.

So I hope you'll take the time to explore a little the inner workings of Chinese medicine. It can bring a great deal of joy and healing into your life.

WHAT IS CHINESE MEDICINE?

Chinese medicine is a 4,000-year-old system of balancing the body's own health-preserving forces. It allows you to create optimum conditions for maintaining and restoring wellness by using the powers of your unified mind/body/spirit. This approach can create self-healing opportunities not available through Western medicine.

HOW A CHINESE MEDICINE DOCTOR VIEWS THE BODY

To a Chinese medicine doctor the body is but one part of the whole human being: Mind/body/spirit is a unit. No Chinese practitioner would ever examine your body without also considering the state of your spirit and your mind—in fact, it couldn't be done. Each of these fundamental aspects of human existence is part of the other; no single one can exist separately nor can it escape the influence of the other aspects. This means that anything that causes upset in one may trigger upset in the others: Disharmony in the Heart Organ System (a possible Western diagnosis might be angina) may trigger mental depression and spiritual malaise. Or a troubled spirit can cause disharmony in the Spleen Organ System, leading to what Western medicine might identify as gastric ulcers. In Chinese medicine, healing can be effective only if treatment addresses the full range of mind/body/spirit problems.

Chinese medicine also has a distinct interpretation of the bodily systems that function within the mind/body/spirit. Unlike Western medicine, which views the body as a composite of analyzable tissues, biochemical reactions, and organ and glandular functions, Chinese medicine views the dynamic life process through the interconnected relationship of *Essential Substances, Organ Systems,* and *channels.* These terms describe the internal working of the mind/body/spirit in ways that are significantly distinct from Western ideas.

Essential Substances

Essential Substances are the fluids, essences, and energies that nurture the Organ Systems and keep the mind/body/spirit in balance. They are identified as Qi, the life force; Shen, the spirit; Jing, the essence; Xue, the blood; and Jin-Ye, additional fluids.

Qi (pronounced CHEE), the Life Force
Qi is quantum energy—both wave and particle, both matter and spirit—that animates being. All life is powered by Qi, which comes in many forms that all work together.

Original Qi, or *Yuan Qi,* enters the body at conception and is stored in the Kidney Organ System. It influences your basic constitution. Disharmony and hard living can use up original Qi.

Grain Qi, or *Gu Qi,* is brought into the body through food and released in the Stomach System.

Air Qi, or *Kong Qi,* is extracted by the Lungs from air we breath.

Normal Qi, or *Zheng Qi,* is what we generally mean when we talk about Qi. It is the result of the combination of Air, Grain, and Original Qi and is important because it creates all body movement; protects the body from disharmony (disease); changes food into Xue (pronounced sh-WHEY; blood), Qi, and fluids such as tears, urine, and sweat.

Organ Qi, or *Zang-Fu Zhi Qi,* makes sure that all your Organ Systems function properly.

Channel Qi, or *Jing Luo Zhi Qi,* moves through the channels to the Organ Systems and links the Organ Systems to the Xue (blood). Acupuncture manipulates Channel Qi.

Nutritive Qi, or *Ying Qi,* creates Xue (blood) by helping the Spleen change food into Xue and moves the Xue through the channels so it can nourish the body.

Protective Qi, or *Wei Qi,* resists and combats external causes of disharmony (disease) that are called Pernicious Influences. It also regulates the sweat glands and pores, moistens and protects skin and hair, and helps the Organs maintain an appropriate warmth.

Ancestral Qi, Pectoral Qi, or *Zong Qi,* is responsible for breathing, speech, and regulating the heartbeat.

Shen, the Spirit

Shen embodies consciousness, emotions, and thoughts. Shen, or spirit, is as real a part of the makeup of human life as blood or flesh. It comes into the fetus from the parents, and must be nurtured and renewed after birth through healthful, balanced living. Shen contains the emotions and flows through the channels to all Organ Systems—that is why an emotional disturbance can cause disharmony in an Organ System and can disrupt the emotions. Every diagnosis takes into account the health of the Shen, and any remedy for disharmony may involve strengthening the Shen. A practitioner may use acupuncture to balance Shen's passage through the channels, Qi Gong exercises and meditation to produce calm and centeredness, balanced nutrition to feed the Shen, and herbs to heal the spirit.

Jing, the Essence

Jing nurtures growth and development and comes in part from our parents and in part from the food we eat. Jing is the fluid essence that contains the life force, defines our basic constitution, and nurtures growth and development. We inherit Prenatal Jing from our parents and it contributes to the formation of Normal Qi. However, once born we can also acquire Jing through the transformation of food in the Spleen and Stomach Systems. At this point Jing becomes dependent on Qi. In fact, Qi and Jing become intertwined: Qi is Yang; Jing is Yin. *Qi and Jing together create the energy and essence of what it is to be alive.* Throughout the various stages of life from early childhood to puberty and maturity through old age, the amount of available Prenatal Jing declines.

Xue, the Blood

Xue is often called blood, but unlike the Western concept of blood it also contains Qi and Shen and isn't confined to veins and arteries. It also moves through the channels (or meridians) along with Qi. It is best thought of as a river that moves through the blood vessels and the channels to help nourish the Organ Systems. Qi creates and powers Xue while Xue nurtures the Organ Systems that make and regulate Qi. The Organ Systems also maintain Xue: The Spleen Organ System governs Xue, keeping it within its proper pathways; the Heart Organ System rules Xue, keeping it moving in a harmonious flow; the Liver Organ System stores it.

Jin-Ye, Additional Fluids

Jin-Ye is all the fluids that are not included in Xue: sweat, urine, mucus, saliva, and secretions such as bile and gastric acid. Produced by water and the digestion of food, and dependent on the harmonious functioning of the Spleen and Stomach Organ Systems, Jin-Ye, like oil in an engine, keeps the body parts running smoothly. It is essential in maintaining healthy lungs and kidneys.

Organ Systems

Organ Systems define the central organ plus its interaction with the Essential Substances (Qi, Xue, Shen, Jing, Jin-Ye) and channels. An organ system governs specific bodily tissue and emotional states. For example, the Heart System is not only responsible for the circulation of blood and Xue, but also regulates and is in charge of storing Shen (spirit). Throughout this book we capitalize references such as Heart System and Organ System to help remind the reader that these elements of the mind/body/spirit are not synonymous with the Western terms such as heart, cardiovascular system, or organ.

Chinese medicine divides the Organ Systems into two categories: the Zang and the Fu. They are described below.

Zang Organs (Yin)

The Zang Organ Systems are predominantly involved with storing Qi, Xue, and other vital essences. They include the following:

The Kidney System manages metabolism of fluids, as Western medicine also
states, but also acts as the ruler of birth, maturation, reproduction, growth, and regeneration. Bones, teeth, the inner ear, the bone marrow, and the brain are also regulated by this Organ System.

The Spleen System, which creates and controls Xue, is vital in taking the Qi from the food you eat and changing it into Xue and Qi. When the Spleen System is balanced, the digestive tract functions well and Jin-Ye fluids and food energy are distributed harmoniously throughout the body.

The Liver System purifies the Xue and maintains harmonious movement of Qi and Xue through the channels and Organ Systems; it also plays an important role in balancing emotions, helping keep frustration and sudden anger at bay.

The Lung System has great influence over Qi because it takes in Air Qi, which contributes to the formation of Normal Qi. It collects Ancestral Qi in the chest area, where it provides the Heart System with Qi and helps manage the movement of water to the Kidney System and sends water vapor through the body. It also rules the exterior of the body through its relationship with Wei (Protective) Qi, providing disease resistance.

The Heart System is associated with the passage of Xue through the blood vessels and with the storage of Shen. When the Heart System's Qi and Shen are well balanced, the overall spirit is in harmony.

The Pericardium System has no physiological function that separates it from the heart, but it is a distinct Organ System because it helps maintain a balance of Heart Qi. It also acts as the protector of the heart muscle and defends the Heart System against assault by external forces that can cause illness and disharmony.

The Fu Organ Systems (Yang)

The Fu Organ Systems take in food, extract nutrition, and excrete waste.

The Gallbladder System helps digestion by working with the Liver to store and secrete bile into the Large and Small Intestine Systems. Disharmony in the Liver Organ System upsets the Gallbladder, and vice versa.

The Stomach System mulches food into essence and fluids so that the Spleen Organ System can then turn them into Qi and Xue. This system also moves Qi downward and directs waste to the Intestine Systems. The Spleen moves Qi upward; harmony between the Stomach and Spleen is crucial to good health.

The Small Intestine System helps the Stomach System produce Qi and Xue and refines fluids into pure (for use by the mind/body/spirit) and impure (for elimination) substances.

The Large Intestine System moves the impure waste down through the body, extracts water, and produces feces.

The Urinary Bladder System excretes wastewater that comes from the Kidney, Lung, and Intestinal Systems.

The Triple Burner System is said to have a "name without shape," and has no direct corollary in Western medicine. It is divided into three parts, the Upper, Middle, and Lower. The Upper Burner distributes the Qi of water and food throughout the body. The Middle Burner is associated with the Spleen and Stomach Systems, and, according to some practitioners, the Liver System. It's involved with digestion, absorption of Essential Substances, evaporating fluids, and imbuing Xue with Nutritive Qi. The Lower Burner, which the Chinese also refer to as a "drainage ditch," refers to an area below the navel and includes the Kidney, the Large and Small Intestine, Urinary Bladder, and Liver (owing to the location of the acupuncture channel). It governs the elimination of impurities. The Lower Burner helps regulate the Large Intestines and helps the Kidney System process waste.

Channels

Channels, or meridians, are the conduits in the vast aqueduct system that transports the Essential Substances such as Qi to the Organ Systems. They also help the body resist pathogens and reflect symptoms of disease and disharmony. Acupuncture works by using needles to open and close the gates that regulate flow of Essential Substances through the channels. When the flow of Essential Substances is uneven, causing either excess or deficiency in an Organ System, then there is disharmony and disease.

THE CYCLICAL FLOW OF QI

TO THE ORGAN SYSTEMS THROUGH

THE TWELVE REGULAR CHANNELS

The channels and the direction of their flow

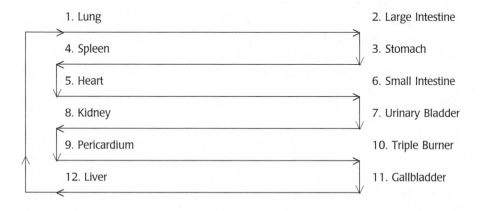

1. Lung	2. Large Intestine
4. Spleen	3. Stomach
5. Heart	6. Small Intestine
8. Kidney	7. Urinary Bladder
9. Pericardium	10. Triple Burner
12. Liver	11. Gallbladder

Each Organ System is paired with another: the Lung and Large Intestine; the Spleen and Stomach; the Heart and Small Intestine; the Kidney and Urinary Bladder; the Pericardium and Triple Burner; and the Liver and Gallbladder. This association means that if one of the paired systems becomes unbalanced, the other may be thrown into disharmony as well.

YIN/YANG

What unifies Essential Substances, Organ Systems, and channels is Yin/Yang, the dynamic balance between opposing forces of creation and destruction. Many Westerners think of Yin/Yang as a symbolic representation of harmony, but in Chinese medicine Yin/Yang is not a simple metaphor—it exists as a palpable force that lives in the body, in Qi, and in the Organ Systems. For example, the Liver, Heart, Spleen, Lung, Kidney, and Pericardium Organ Systems are Yin; the Gallbladder, Small Intestine, Stomach, Large Intestine, Urinary Bladder, and Triple Burner (the Chinese system that governs metabolism) Organ Systems are Yang. When the balance of Yin/Yang is disturbed, disharmony develops. When Yin is disturbed, chronic conditions can take root that produce pain in the body, changes in tongue shape, a deep pulse, and changes in bowel movements or urine. When Yang is disturbed, disharmony can trigger acute chills, fever, body aches, an aversion to cold and wind, a thin coating on the tongue, and what the Chinese call a floating pulse.

When a Chinese medicine doctor perceives a symptom that is Yin or Yang it provides a clue as to where the disease is lodged, what other imbalances it may be causing, and what needs to be done to restore harmony and balance.

HOW CHINESE MEDICINE VIEWS DISEASE

Chinese medicine focuses on the relationships between the parts of the body and the mind/body/spirit. Any disturbance in these relationships, which is a sign of ill health, is described as a *disharmony* or an *imbalance*. There is no discussion of diseases or viruses or infections. You don't come down with pneumonia, you develop a disharmony.

A thousand years ago, if the Chinese had known that viruses and bacteria existed, these would have been included in their understanding of the forces that create ill health. However, they didn't and as a consequence, although modern Chinese medicine practitioners recognize that viruses and bacteria exist, Traditional Chinese Medicine *theory* does not acknowledge the presence of these infectious agents. But Chinese medicine is a pragmatic system, and *therapy* does in fact acknowledge the existence of viruses and bacteria and takes them into account and responds to their presence appropriately.

As a result, in Chinese medicine the goal of treatment is not to cure a disease but to restore harmony in the whole person—mind/body/spirit.

To treat a complaint, the Chinese medicine practitioner focuses on identifying symptoms, understanding what they indicate about the condition of your mind/body/spirit, and restoring optimal function. The emphasis is on results; there is less concern with how or why problems exist or therapies work.

This approach to identifying health problems may make it difficult in the beginning to understand how Chinese medicine practitioners describe HIV disease and related syndromes. For example, if you seek treatment for a common yeast infection, such as candidiasis, the practitioner may offer treatments for disharmonies described as Spleen Qi Deficiency, Dampness (Hot or Cold), and possibly stagnant Liver Qi. The therapies prescribed (herbs, acupuncture, dietary changes, Qi Gong exercise, and meditation) will be designed to rebalance the Essential Elements and Organ Systems. When balance is restored, the symptoms—in this case what Western medicine calls candidiasis—will go away.

WHAT IS HEALING?

Chinese medicine reharmonizes the mind/body/spirit, and that allows a person to heal his or her physical, mental, and psychic wounds, even when a cure, in the Western sense, is not attainable.

How is this possible?

Acupuncture, herbs, Qi Gong, and dietary therapy do more than address specific maladies or diseases. They allow people to achieve a peaceful resolution of stress, an unaggressive yet masterful acceptance of responsibility for their own well-being. This in turn helps them find a wholeness, to heal pain. That is what eases the overall disharmony that is so often associated with chronic and life-threatening diseases, and makes a person feel whole.

But Chinese medicine's view of disease and manner of treatment is as practical as conventional Western therapies. The two fundamental principles of Chinese medicine that apply to management of infectious diseases such as HIV/AIDS are called Fu Zheng and Jiedu/Qiuxie: Fu Zheng uses treatments to strengthen the body's natural disease-fighting systems (i.e., the immune system). Jiedu/Qiuxie focuses on eliminating External Pernicious Influences (outside pathogens). In addition, over the millennia a lot of clinical work has gone into handling disharmonies that trigger deficiencies and lead to wasting and exhaustion, conditions that also are associated with HIV/AIDS.

In Western terms, Fu Zheng and Jiedu/Qiuxie would be called immune-regulating and antitoxin therapies. They offer treatments to alleviate metabolic changes that trigger night sweats, low-grade fever, and weight loss, and they counter what are called opportunistic infections, such as pneumonia and thrush.

HOW THIS AFFECTS THE WAY MEDICINE IS PRACTICED

The Diagnostic Process

The diagnostic process in Chinese medicine involves looking for signs of disharmony by going through what is called the Four Examinations: Inquiring,

Looking, Listening/Smelling (in Chinese these are related processes), and Touching.

Inquiring centers around questions on your reaction to heat and cold, your patterns of perspiration, if and when you experience headaches or dizziness; what type of pain, if any, you may have; your bowel and bladder functions; your thirst, appetite, and tastes; sleep patterns; sexual functioning; sexual activity and reproductive history; general medical history; general physical activity; and emotions.

Looking involves examination of the tongue, body language, and facial color. The coating, color, and shape of the tongue give clues as to the specific location of internal disharmony. For example, a wet and heavily coated tongue (said to have excess fur) may indicate excess Jin-Ye—an excess of fluids, which can signal disharmony in the Spleen System's ability to move fluids. Body language also reveals the condition of the mind/body/spirit. For example, a person who has a soft voice, hesitant gestures, and sits with his arms wrapped around his torso may have a deficiency and an imbalance of Qi. Facial color gives the practitioner additional clues to the nature and severity of internal disharmony: a light yellow pallor indicates that the Spleen System is damp and cold, a condition that may trigger diarrhea. Dark yellow indicates Damp Heat, a different cause of diarrhea.

Listening/Smelling involves evaluating the quality of the voice and general odor. An excess condition is indicated if a person's voice is loud; a deficiency if the voice is low and weak. When combined with other subtle observations, a practitioner can develop a more specific diagnosis. For example, if someone suffers from the blues, sounds apathetic, and has chilly hands and pale urine, then deficient Qi and cold may be indicated. The practitioner also makes note of how the person smells, his breath and general body odor. If someone emits a strong stench from secretions or excretions, that may indicate the disharmony is caused by excess Heat; a weaker odor may indicate that a Cold Deficiency is at work.

Touching is done by reading the pulse and by pressing on acupuncture points along the channels to see if that triggers or eases pain.

Pulse reading is a complicated process that involves careful discrimination among 28 different rhythms and qualities. For example, your practitioner may say your pulse is floating, slippery, choppy, wiry, tight, slow, rapid, thin, big, empty, or full. Each one of these pulse types is associated with specific disharmonies.

Palpation of the acupuncture points along the channels and on the abdomen helps a practitioner determine if your Essential Substances (Qi, Xue, Jing, Shen, and Jin-Ye) are working harmoniously or if there is a disharmony affecting one or more of them. (Abdominal palpation is central to the practice of Japanese acupuncture.)

Once these factors are evaluated, the doctor is ready to move toward a diagnosis. Depending on your symptoms the doctor will decide if any of the Essential Substances are excess, deficient, or stagnant. She will determine what Organ Systems are affected. Then it is time to prescribe an individualized set of therapies to help the mind/body/spirit restore harmony and balance to the system.

Healing Techniques

Once the diagnosis is complete, practitioners may prescribe one or more of four basic healing techniques: dietary therapy, herbal therapy, acupuncture and moxibustion, and Qi Gong exercise/meditation. A brief description follows here, and each therapy is discussed in detail in Chapters 6–9.

Acupuncture and Moxibustion

Acupuncture controls the flow of Qi through the channels by using needles inserted at specific points to control the opening and closing of gates along the channels. If there is excess in some area, a gate is opened so that the pool of essential substances can circulate more freely; if there is a deficiency the gates are closed so that area of the body can retain sufficient essential substances to become restored to balance.

Moxibustion is the use of a heated herb (usually mugwort), placed on or near a specific acupuncture point to stimulate the flow of Qi. I believe this is an essential element of treatment in HIV disease—more significant than acupuncture itself.

Acupressure and channel massage are based on the same principles as acupuncture, and use pressure to stimulate the flow of Qi in the channels.

Dietary Therapy

Chinese medicine is founded in part on the belief that you are what you eat. Food not only influences the quality of Qi, the health of Organ Systems, and your moods, it can also be used as a therapy for disharmonies and disorders. A Chinese medicine protocol often begins with dietary therapy.

Chinese Herbal Medicine

Chinese herbs are powerful medicine, and for the most part should be taken only under the direction of a trained herbalist. They are used singly and in combination to reestablish harmony in the mind/body/spirit. Despite the name, not all "herbal" medicine comes from plants; in the Chinese pharmacopoeia are medicinal substances derived from mineral and animal products as well.

Qi Gong Exercise/Meditation

Qi Gong, the Chinese art of exercise and meditation, combines movement, still postures, and meditation to influence the flow of Qi. It is an effective way to strengthen disease resistance, ease stress, and restore harmony to troubled Organ Systems.

This about covers the basic principles of Chinese medicine. Let's turn our attention to how Chinese and Western medicine view disease and resistance to disease, and HIV infection in particular.

PART II

Guardians
of Harmony:

*The Immune System in
Chinese and Western Medicine*

Chinese and Western medical treatments are derived from two distinct approaches to scientific inquiry and from sharply contrasting ways of analyzing and describing the dynamics of disease. Yet each provides a clear picture of certain aspects of what it means to maintain wellness and struggle against unwellness: The West sees the complex cellular activity that characterizes the immune system; the East sees the interrelationship of all aspects of mind/body/spirit and the role they play in resisting disharmony. Together these perspectives offer a comprehensive view of how to most effectively maintain health and fight illness.

3

Maintaining Balance:
The Chinese View of the Body's
Ability to Fight Disease

In treating illness, it is necessary to examine the entire context,
scrutinize the symptoms, observe the emotions and attitudes.
—*The Nei Jing, the Inner Classic of the Yellow Emperor:*
Simple Questions (Translated by Ted Kaptchuk)

In Chinese medicine, the body's battle against disease is fought on two levels—superficially, at skin level, through the vigilance of Protective Qi, and inside the body through the harmonious functioning of the Organ Systems and the Essential Substances. These two aspects of the "immune system" work both separately and together to form a protective network that responds to external and internal assaults on the mind/body/spirit.

This highly responsive defense system is called upon to combat three types of disease triggers:

- *The External Pernicious Influences,* identified as climatic factors of heat, cold, wind, dampness, dryness, and Summer Heat.
- *The Epidemic Factors,* nonclimatic External Pernicious Influences that are often infectious and attack deep within the body, bypassing the Protective Qi and causing disruption in Organ Systems almost immediately.
- *The Internal Disharmonies,* which are associated with Organ System imbalances and with disharmony of the Seven Emotions—joy, anger, fear and fright, sadness, and grief and worry—that can precipitate disease from within the body.

THE BATTLE AGAINST EXTERNAL PERNICIOUS INFLUENCES

Sometimes, a Pernicious Influence breaches the perimeter patrolled by Wei (Protective) Qi and enters the body. This can happen if it is simply so powerful that it overwhelms the Wei Qi, or because your mind/body/spirit is already weakened by chronic exhaustion, poor diet, stress, or sadness, for example, or you don't have enough inherent constitutional strength to fight off the in-vader. Once an External Pernicious Influence gets around the defenses of Wei (Protective) Qi, you develop a disharmony.

UNDERSTANDING THE TERMINOLOGY

In Chinese medicine, when you are ill you are said to have a "disharmony" or an "imbalance." These are interchangeable terms used to describe a whole complex of interrelated symptoms and syndromes affecting the mind/body/spirit. The nature of a disharmony is determined by its impact on the condition of the Essential Substances, Organ Systems, and channels.

In Western medicine, the term "disease" usually connotes a narrow concept: the unified set of symptoms that result from a single cause. The concept of *disease complex* is more equivalent to the concept of disharmony. For example, when talking about the disease complex related to HIV/AIDS, Western doctors are describing an interrelated package of syndromes and diseases of the digestive tract, skin, neural system, and much more—and they are recognizing the potential involvement of fluids, muscles, nerves, mental functions, and many other components of the body. At the same time, they acknowledge that any individual infected with HIV may experience the various symptoms in a highly individual pattern and with individual repercussions. This is very much how a Chinese medicine practitioner thinks about disharmony. It is here, on the frontier of Western understanding of immune dysfunction, that Eastern and Western medical thought come closest together.

External Cold

These illnesses are generally acute, with chills, fever, and achy joints. When they strike, symptoms include a fear of cold and headaches. With External Cold, putting on warm clothes or blankets will not warm you up because the cold is trapped near the surface of the body in the skin. The only way to remove the chill is to stimulate the Wei (Protective) Qi so it expels the cold from the surface through the use of herbs and acupuncture. If the External Cold moves to the interior, you may experience lethargy, grogginess, craving for heat, loose stools, clear draining sinuses, and develop a pale tongue.

External Heat

These disorders often cause a red face, hyperactivity and talkativeness, fever, and a rapid pulse. You may also experience sweating and severe sore throat. The tongue's coating is yellow. When the heat penetrates deeper into the body you may become thirsty or constipated or develop rashes. If the heat attacks the Shen (spirit) you may become delirious and your speech may become confused or slurred.

Related to the External Pernicious Influence Heat, Toxic Heat is a particularly virulent infectious condition that is identified as an Epidemic Factor. The Chinese medicine text, *Discussion of Warm Epidemics,* written in 1642, recognizes the existence of Pestilences—called *li qi* or *yi qi.* These are diseases that are not caused by the climatic factors of heat, cold, wind, dampness, dryness, or Summer Heat, but by external infectious agents. And they often trigger symptoms that are similar to the External Pernicious Influence Heat, but are severely toxic because they strike directly at the interior of the body. In fact, they seem to scoot around Protective Qi altogether. HIV, which is transmitted only through exchange of fluids, is an example of this type of attack on the body's inner harmony.

External Dampness

This can invade the body and the channels and block the smooth flow of Qi, causing stiff joints and heavy limbs. When dampness penetrates more deeply, a person can develop nausea, loss of appetite, bloating, and/or diarrhea. As External Dampness moves to the interior, it is associated with bodily secretions and can lead to tumors, coughing, and, if it invades the Shen (spirit), to erratic behavior and insanity. Once Dampness has settled in, it is hard to displace.

External Dryness

This is often coupled with heat, but unlike heat alone, which produces redness and warmth, dryness and heat create evaporation and cracking. When dryness invades the body you may develop respiratory problems such as asthma, dry skin, or a dry, hacking cough.

Summer Heat

This is always associated with exposure to extreme heat and it wracks the whole body, causing a sudden high fever and complete exhaustion, reminiscent of heat stroke. It is often accompanied by dampness.

External Wind

This is often joined with an invasion of cold or heat and is associated with tics, twitches, fear of drafts, headaches, and a stuffed-up nose.

Once a Pernicious Influence penetrates the defensive layer maintained by Wei (Protective) Qi and begins to make you sick, you want to act quickly to help the body reestablish harmony. This is done through the use of herbs, acupuncture, dietary therapy, and Qi Gong exercise and meditation; they regulate Qi and other Essential Substances and reharmonize the working of the individual Organ Systems.

However, if balance and optimal functioning cannot be restored, the Pernicious Influence may penetrate deeper into the body. This makes the disharmony more severe and the symptoms more difficult to treat. For more detailed information see my first book, *The Chinese Way to Healing: Many Paths to Wholeness* (Perigee Books, 1996).

WHICH PERNICIOUS INFLUENCES AFFECT YOU MOST OFTEN?

Most people find that they are more vulnerable to either heat or cold and that dampness or dryness is most affecting. For example, those who have constitutions that make them susceptible to the negative influences of heat may find that they experience more symptoms of External Heat than of any of the other Pernicious Influences. After reviewing the descriptions of the Pernicious Influences in this section, would you say you are more affected by heat or cold? Dampness or dryness? Summer heat? Wind?

THE BATTLE AGAINST INTERNAL DISHARMONIES

There are times when disharmonies develop not because of External Pernicious Influences or Epidemic Factors, but because of internal imbalances in the Organ Systems, the Essential Substances, or the Seven Emotions (explained below).

Internal imbalances in the Organ Systems and Essential Substances occur because of poor nutrition, stress and overexertion, inharmonious sexual activity, trauma both physical and emotional, parasites and poisons, and/or a weak constitution.

Poor Nutrition

Diet has an enormous impact on the well-being of the mind/body/spirit. Nutritional excesses or deficiencies have a negative impact on the Stomach and Spleen Systems, which are responsible for receiving and changing food into Qi and Xue and other Essential Substances. Once these organ systems are affected, many associated functions get thrown out of whack as well.

Stress and Overexertion

Expending energy, even in a harmonious way, consumes Qi. Overexertion—too much exercise, overwork, emotional turmoil—depletes Qi more severely. Since overwork and stressful lifestyles are often associated with bad eating habits—skipped meals, fast foods, excess alcohol consumption, and cigarette smoking—the problems are compounded. This inevitably leads to disruption of all of the Organ Systems, especially the Stomach, Spleen, Liver, and Kidney.

Inharmonious Sexual Activity

Excessive, discordant, or emotionally or physically disruptive sex can cause deficiency disorders, especially in men. There is no absolute measure of what constitutes inharmonious or excessive sex—one person's constitution may be more affected than another's by the same activities. Whatever constitutes unhealthy sex for you, the associated symptoms are profound fatigue, lower-back problems, frequent urination, even dizziness and weak knees. In traditional Chinese medicine texts it is recommended that sexual activity be regulated by age and season: Men at the age of 15 *in good health* may enjoy sex twice a day; at 30, once a day; at 40, every three days; at 50, every five days; and at 60, every ten days. When there is deficient Qi or disharmony in the Kidney, frequency should be reduced. Sexual activity should increase in the spring and decrease in the winter.

Excess sexual activity in women is viewed slightly differently than in men. Men are depleted through ejaculation (that's why many HIV-positive men practice Tantric sex, which teaches you how to conserve Qi through withholding ejaculation when you have an orgasm), and men's sexual energy is related to Kidney Jing (essence); some texts say women are depleted through orgasm and their sexual energy is associated with Xue (blood). However, it is generally agreed that in women, bearing too many children in too short a time depletes Kidney essence and that's why there is a correlation between excess childbirth in women and excess sexual activity in men.

Trauma

Physical trauma creates Qi and Xue Stagnation in the area that is injured. In Chinese medicine the impact of a localized trauma is understood to persist after the pain or bruise goes away. The stagnation can cause long-term problems in the channels and associated Organ Systems that must be reharmonized so that recurrent problems don't arise. Scars, even after healing, may block the channels or allow Qi to "leak" from them for years after the injury or surgery.

Parasites and Poisons

Although fungal infections and parasites enter the body from the outside, Chinese medicine considers diet a contributing factor. If your diet is heavy in fatty or sweet foods, it can produce dampness, which offers parasites a fertile environment in which to reproduce.

Weak Constitution

As we've discussed, we are all born with a supply of Prenatal Qi and Jing, which we receive from our parents while we are in the womb. If our parents are in poor health at the time of conception, we won't get the ample supply of

Qi and Jing we need to become a strong person. Smoking and drinking during pregnancy also may lead to a weak constitution in the child. Although it is difficult, you can improve your basic constitution by strengthening it with proper diet and Qi Gong exercise and through acupuncture and herbal treatments.

LOOKING INSIDE

Now it's time to take a moment to reflect on your lifestyle habits and their impact on your physical, spiritual, and emotional well-being. Do you eat well? Are you prone to overexercise? Review your sexual activity. Does it feel harmonious or out of balance? As you work to restore harmony to all your systems, you will explore these issues more deeply: For example, in the program for managing chronic diarrhea you will do an extensive analysis of your dietary habits. But it's important to begin to tune in to the connection between how you live and how you heal.

Internal Disharmonies Associated with the Seven Emotions

Well-balanced emotions and peaceful spirituality are considered important cornerstones of the body's defense against disharmony and disease. Any time an emotion becomes too inflamed or suppressed, it can affect the balance of Qi and other Essential Substances and the Organ Systems. And because the emotions are internal triggers of disharmony, they tend to affect the mind/body/spirit quite deeply and are often difficult to treat. The Seven Emotions' (anger, joy, sadness, grief, worry, fear, fright) targets of disharmony are the following:

The Liver System. The Liver System, which governs the Xue (blood) and emotions, is the organ system most commonly affected by inharmonious or disturbed emotions, and is especially vulnerable to anger and repressed feelings.

The Heart System. The Heart System, which stores Shen (spirit), is upset by too much or too little joy. Some practitioners advise their clients with HIV disease not to read newspapers or magazine articles on AIDS because so often the reports are negative and that can create disharmony in the Heart System in those who are particularly sensitive.

Symptoms associated with emotion-triggered Heart System disharmonies include insomnia, fuzzy thinking, laughing and crying jags, and, when particularly severe, hysteria and even madness.

The Lung System. Since it is associated with bringing in and letting go, the Lung System is particularly susceptible to disharmonies triggered by sadness and grief. This translates into an inability to move past traumas or sadness. It's especially important in the management of HIV/AIDS because there is so much grief and sadness, both individually and collectively, in communities highly affected by HIV disease.

The Spleen System. Those who dwell too deeply on their worries or who skip over them in denial can upset the system's balance and this can trigger anxiety and lack of concentration. The constant fixation on specific worries—for example, unremitting worry about being sick with HIV disease—can lead to loose stools and trouble handling the mental demands of a job.

The Kidney System. Fear and fright may trigger disturbances in this system. Furthermore, Kidney disturbances are often associated with the exercise of or lack of ability to exercise the will, which often happens to people who are overwhelmed by the difficulties associated with managing a life-threatening chronic illness.

Symptoms of Internal Disharmonies

Regardless of whether your internal disharmony is triggered by a weak constitution, inharmonious sex, or an obsession with food from a drive-through window, it is likely to fall into one of five categories: Internal Cold, Internal Heat, Internal Dampness, Internal Dryness, and Internal Wind.

Internal Cold is associated with diarrhea, feeling cold, lethargy, a pale tongue, fatigue, and slowing down of body processes. It is characterized by feeling warmer when you bundle up (unlike with External Cold), and craving warm drinks. You may sleep for extended periods of time, perhaps curled up in a fetal position. Any pains you have may be eased by the application of warmth.

Internal Heat is associated with feeling hot and with hyperactivity. You may talk too much, crave cold drinks, and have a rapid pulse and a red tongue. Secretions become thick and dark, with a strong smell.

Internal Dampness is associated with nausea, lack of appetite, diarrhea, tumors, coughing, bloating, and edema. You may have a swollen tongue or thick tongue fur.

Internal Dryness manifests as asthma, a dry cough, and dry skin. You may be constipated, feel parched. When dryness is combined with a heat condition, you will develop redness.

Internal Wind creates twitches, headaches, seizures, and dizziness. It can also produce symptoms such as pain, rashes, itchiness, or numbness that move from one spot to another in the body. For example, one day you may have a headache on the left side of your head; the next it is on the right side.

HOW CHINESE MEDICINE DESCRIBES DISHARMONIES: THE EIGHT FUNDAMENTAL PATTERNS

Now that we've seen the kinds of disharmonies that exist in Chinese medicine, we can take a quick look at the Eight Fundamental Patterns, which describe the character of the disharmonies. The eight patterns are interior, exterior, heat, cold, excess, deficient, Yin and Yang. They describe the way a disharmony and disease have affected the Organ Systems and Essential Substances. The eight patterns are also used to describe the dynamic balance between Yin and Yang within the mind/body/spirit.

Interior and *exterior* describe the location of a disharmony in the body. Exterior disharmonies are often acute and are associated with chills, fever, an aversion to cold, and an allover achy feeling. Interior disharmonies may cause changes in bowel movements and in urination, and discomfort or pain in the trunk of the body. They are also associated with the lack of aversion to cold or wind.

Heat and *cold* describe the state of activity of the body and the nature of the disease. Cold patterns are caused by deficient Yang or a Cold External Pernicious Influence. With cold everything slows down and a person becomes withdrawn and sleeps in a curled-up position. Pain is relieved by warmth, bodily secretions are thin and clear, and there is a desire for warm liquids.

Heat patterns are caused by the invasion of the External Pernicious Influence Heat, the depletion of Yin substances—through dehydration, for example—and excess Yang. With heat, the body's processes speed up and a person may talk excessively, have a red face and hot body, and prefer cold beverages; secretions become thick, putrid, and dark.

Deficiency and *excess* are used to describe the impact of the disharmony on the body's Normal Qi.

A person with a deficiency may feel weak and tentative, have a pale or ashen complexion, sweat easily, have problems with incontinence, breathe shallowly, and experience pain that decreases with pressure. When an Organ System has a Qi Deficiency it is underactive and weak.

A person with an excess condition may demonstrate heavy forceful movements, a loud full voice, heavy breathing, and pain that increases with pressure. When an Organ System is afflicted with an excess pattern of disharmony it is sluggish and unresponsive. A chronic excess condition leads to stagnation. Essential Substances are often said to be stagnant.

Yin and *Yang*, when used to describe a pattern of disharmony, encompass the other six Fundamental Patterns. Yin encompasses interior, cold, and deficient; Yang encompasses exterior, heat, and excess.

Diagnosing a disharmony as Yin or Yang depends on first ascertaining the presence of other fundamental patterns. For example, during diagnosis, a Chinese medicine practitioner will first try to figure out where the disharmony is located, on the interior or the exterior. Then the practitioner will search for symptoms that reveal whether the disharmony is acting as though it were a pattern of heat or cold, excess or deficiency. For example, if the practitioner observes the patient's disharmony is exhibiting symptoms of the patterns heat and excess—fast, forceful movements and pain that is intensified by pressure and soothed by cold—then the diagnosis will be a Heat Excess Yang disorder.

HOW DISEASE IMPACTS THE ESSENTIAL SUBSTANCES

The Essential Substances develop disharmonies as a result of Pernicious Influences, Epidemic Factors, and disrupted emotions. As mentioned above, those disharmonies conform to specific patterns: interior and exterior; excess and deficiency; heat and cold; Yin and Yang. Those patterns affect the Essential Substances—Qi, Xue (blood), Jing, Jin-Ye, and Shen (spirit)—in specific ways, triggering symptoms. Let's look at how those patterns are described.

Qi May Become Excess, Stagnant, or Deficient

• When Qi does not flow smoothly through the channels and the Organ Systems, but pools up, some areas of the body end up with excess Qi and others with deficient Qi. This can happen because of the invasion of a Pernicious Influence, the suppression of an emotion, poor nutrition, or even a traumatic injury.

Symptoms may include pain that worsens with pressure and is not easy to locate precisely; frequently the pain comes and goes in response to your emotions. You may also experience bloating and belching, achiness all over, and fidgetiness.

• Frequently, excess Qi collects and becomes *stagnant.* Severe stagnant Qi can, in turn, become rebellious, leading to hiccups, vomiting, coughing, asthma, liver problems, and fainting.

• Deficient Qi happens when poor nutrition, lack of exercise, respiration problems, and/or disharmony of the spirit and mind use up Qi and don't replenish it. This can lead to spontaneous sweating, fatigue, lethargy and weakness, a weak voice, a pale but bright face, disharmony of a particular Organ System, and symptoms that become worse when you move around.

When severe, deficient Qi can evolve into collapsed or sinking Qi, which is characterized by Organ prolapse, vertigo, weariness, and a very weak pulse.

Shen May Become Disturbed or Deficient

There are two types of Shen disharmonies: disturbed Shen and deficient Shen. These are both triggered by disharmony in one of the seven internal emotions and may be accompanied by stagnant Qi and disharmony in the Heart and the Liver Organ Systems. Sometimes, if the Heart has a Xue (blood) Deficiency, the Spleen System may also be involved. Feeling out of sorts, fatigued, blue, grumpy, and dispirited—the classic indications of a developing Shen disharmony—is often the first sign of a developing sickness or disorder.

• Disturbed Shen is associated with forgetfulness, disorientation, trouble sleeping, and a dull look in the eyes. If it becomes severe, profound mental instability may develop.

• Lack of Shen makes a person physically unresponsive and verbally uncommunicative.

Xue (blood) May Become Either Deficient or Excess

• Deficient Xue may arise because of malnutrition, blood loss, deficiency in the Spleen Organ System, lack of sufficient Qi, and emotional stress. Symptoms include sleeplessness, dry skin, dizziness, hair loss, palpitations, menstrual irregularities, and blurry vision. In addition, lack of sufficient Xue in the Organ Systems can cause secondary disharmonies and severe Xue Deficiency, affecting the whole body and causing dry skin and a sallow complexion.

• Excess Xue often results from tissue trauma, such as cuts, bruises, and abrasions, or from stagnant Qi, deficient Xue, or cold-obstructing Xue. Symptoms include stabbing, fixed pain, tumors, or swollen organs.

Jing Tends to Become Deficient

We're born with our lifetime supply of Jing, the fluidlike essence that is essential for reproduction and development, and we deplete it bit by bit as we age, as we neglect ourselves, as we battle stress and tension. Although it can be replenished, this takes some effort. That's why we all tend toward Jing Deficiency as we age.

• Symptoms of deficient Jing may include congenital disabilities, improper maturation, premature aging, sexual problems, and infertility. Jing disharmonies are associated with a deficient Kidney System.

Jin-Ye May Be Either Deficient or Excess

Jin-Ye, the bodily fluids—other than Xue (blood)—such as urine and sweat, can also be easily used up through poor nutrition and other destructive personal habits. Sometimes when dampness invades, excess Jin-Ye may become a problem.

• Symptoms of deficient Jin-Ye include lack of moisture in skin, lips, hair, and eyes.

• Symptoms of excess Jin-Ye include stagnation of fluids, edema, and swelling.

HOW DISEASE IMPACTS THE
ORGAN SYSTEMS AND THE CHANNELS

The Organ Systems and the channels are also subject to disharmonies when attacked by External Pernicious Influences or disturbed by the internal Seven Emotions, and those disharmonies conform to the Eight Fundamental Patterns described above. However, because there are so many and the descriptions are a bit long, we have decided not to include them in this book. When your Chinese medicine practitioner makes a diagnosis, I urge you to refer to *The Chinese Way to Healing* to find out what symptoms are associated with it.

This completes our preliminary exploration of the Chinese medicine concepts of health and of disharmony. Now let's take a look at the Chinese view of HIV/AIDS and associated disorders and diseases.

4

❋

Toxic Heat, Spleen/Stomach Deficiency, and the Human Immunodeficiency Virus: HIV Disease from the Chinese Perspective

> When I was first diagnosed I couldn't come to terms with the disease.
> I didn't know how to think about it and what it was doing to me.
> But when I started getting Chinese medicine treatments my
> relationship to my body changed, and my attitude about the disease
> changed. The Chinese medicine description of the disease gave me a
> way to think about my health and my healing and to take charge of
> my medical care.
> —Stephanie, 43, a former computer programmer, diagnosed in 1991

As early as the fifth century B.C., the *Nei Jing*, a classic Chinese medical text, discussed treatments for a complex of syndromes characterized as *xu lao*, or "disease of weakness," and *lao zhai*, "consumptive exhaustion." Looking at the text now, with a Western knowledge of the immune system, I'm amazed by how these syndromes describe disharmonies that sound a lot like the problems we associate with immune dysfunction and HIV/AIDS. Although HIV/AIDS itself did not exist thousands of years ago, the Chinese syndromes associated with HIV/AIDS are related to syndromes described in the *Nei Jing*. At that time, practitioners associated those disharmonies with drug addiction (alcohol), immoderate sexual practices, and poor hygiene.[1]

WHAT TRIGGERS HIV DISEASE?

Through clinical observation and treatment of thousands of people with HIV and AIDS, clinical evaluation of the tongues of over 600 people with HIV infection and/or AIDS, and the use of pulse diagnosis, I have come to understand that HIV infection is triggered by Toxic Heat, and initially attacks the Spleen and Stomach Organ Systems. They are the central organs involved in this complex syndrome and must be supported throughout the entire course of the disease, even when the HIV-related disharmonies expand to involve all the other Organ Systems as well.

THE IMPACT OF TOXIC HEAT

Toxic Heat creates the initial flulike symptoms that for many people accompany initial exposure to HIV. As the Toxic Heat moves more deeply into all systems of the body, it triggers a whole variety of common HIV-related symptoms: pruritis (chronic itching), sore throat, increase in body temperature, feeling as though you always have a fever even if none is present, a nagging sensation that something toxic is present in the body.

Toxic Heat is also responsible for the cascade of Organ System disharmonies in the Spleen and Stomach, Kidney, and Liver, which contribute to the major complication associated with HIV infection, wasting.

THE ROLE OF THE SPLEEN AND STOMACH SYSTEMS IN THE PROGRESSION FROM HIV TO AIDS

The Spleen and Stomach Systems govern the digestive process, transforming food energy and fluid into Qi and Xue (blood). As a result, the Spleen and Stomach moisten and nurture all the other Organ Systems and channels.

When Toxic Heat disrupts the Spleen and Stomach Systems, it triggers symptoms that are associated with the very early stages of HIV infection. These symptoms include

- Fatigue
- Inability to gain weight, no matter how much is eaten
- Loose stools
- Bloating, gas and flatulence, and/or dull pain in the abdomen
- Need to take naps after meals
- Frequent infections

In addition, symptoms of early-stage HIV infection, such as dry skin and lips, set in when the flow of fluids and food essence from the Spleen and Stomach to the Lungs is disrupted. Often, dryness in one area triggers dampness in another: Spleen Qi Deficiency with dampness manifests in early neuropathy (a numbness or tingling sensation, often in the hands or feet), lymphadenopathy (swelling and inflammation of the lymph nodes), vaginal candidiasis (yeast) infections, more serious loose stools, and/or bloating. Spleen-related diarrhea is prevalent with loose stools and abdominal bloating after eating. Skin rashes, commonly associated with early-stage HIV infection, are a result of Spleen Qi Deficiency and Lung disharmonies interacting with the Essential Substances.

Spleen Qi Deficiency also causes deficient Xue (blood). Once this sets in, the door is opened for Toxic Heat to enter the depleted blood and penetrate ever deeper into the body. The body then moves into more advanced stages of HIV/AIDS. If unchecked, an increasing depletion of the fluids of the Spleen (the Spleen's Yin aspect) leads to overall Yin Deficiency, which in turn can lead to Yang depletion. When the spleen becomes deficient, wasting becomes severe. Diarrhea stops. The skin becomes drier and drier. Thirst is unquenchable. Fevers spike every afternoon and often in the evenings. The pulse is rapid, thready, and superficial.

The combination of Western and Chinese therapies can arrest the progression of HIV infection to end-stage AIDS for some period of time. However, when the cascade of Spleen-Stomach–triggered disorders causes overall Yin Deficiency and Yang depletion, a person enters a terminal stage of AIDS. Acupuncture and herbs are then used to support the Shen (spirit) and to ease the passing over to a new phase of existence.

ASSOCIATED DISHARMONIES AND OPPORTUNISTIC INFECTIONS

Toxic Heat and the Spleen-Stomach disharmonies weaken the body's overall resistance to assault from both internal and external disease factors and allow other Organ Systems to become involved. This leads to the development of HIV-related disorders and opportunistic infections. For example, if Toxic Heat assaults the Lungs, PCP (*Pneumocystis carinii* pneumonia) may develop. Xue disharmonies are associated with Kaposi's sarcoma (a proliferative circulatory-cell disease that causes skin lesions); dampness is associated with candidiasis (yeast infections) and fungal invasions; Yin Deficiency and Xue Deficiency are associated with MAC (*Mycobacterium avium* complex); dampness and Spleen and Lung disharmonies may manifest as chronic sinusitis; disturbed Shen is associated with mental disturbances that accompany HIV/AIDS; and many more.

Each of these syndromes is detailed in the individual treatment programs in Part IV. However, I wanted to make the point here that looking at HIV disease as an assault by Toxic Heat that starts with damage to the Spleen and Stomach and moves on to include other Organ Systems and Essential Substances provides a concise method of describing, diagnosing, and treating the whole constellation of HIV-related diseases.

SOME EXAMPLES OF CHINESE MEDICINE HIV/AIDS
DIAGNOSES AND SYMPTOMS

Chinese Medicine HIV/AIDS Syndromes	Signs and Symptoms
Toxic Heat	High fevers; delirium; severe itching
Spleen Qi Deficiency	Diarrhea; frequent infections; loss of appetite; weight loss; nausea; dull pain and bloating in abdomen; gas and flatulence
Spleen Yang Deficiency	Always cold (especially hands and feet); constant watery diarrhea with undigested food; slow pulse and scalloped tongue
Kidney Qi Deficiency	Swollen legs; inability to urinate; pale and swollen tongue
Kidney Yang Deficiency	Cold in Middle/Lower Burners; early-morning diarrhea; low-back pain; extreme fatigue; slow, deep, and thready pulse; pale and swollen tongue
Kidney Yin Deficiency	Night sweats; low-back pain; afternoon and evening fevers; restlessness; chronic sore throat; swollen lymph glands; thready rapid pulse or superficial big and weak pulse (Yang is leaving body)
Liver Qi Stagnation	Irritability; depression; premenstrual syndrome; full feeling in flanks and abdomen; gas and flatulence
Liver Yang rising	Flushing up; hot sensation in chest; headaches
Lung Qi Deficiency	Cough; shortness of breath with little exertion; fatigue; thready weak pulse; pale tongue
Lung Yin Deficiency	Dry cough; coughing blood; afternoon fever; night sweats; hot palms, soles, and chest; red cheeks; itchy skin

Chinese Medicine HIV/AIDS Syndromes	Signs and Symptoms
Shen disturbance	Disorientation; insomnia; dream-disturbed sleep; inability to communicate
Xue Deficiency	Fatigue; sallow face; thready and weak pulse; pale tongue; pale face; pale nails; anemia
Xue Stagnation	Purple spots; severe, stabbing pain

5

The War Within:
Western Immunology and HIV

It is not the purpose or intention of this book to provide you with an in-depth explanation of the Western science of immunology. I do want to acquaint you with the basics of the immune system, however, so that you can appreciate the differences between the Chinese and Western views on the origins and treatment of disease and begin to appreciate how well they complement each other. The most powerful medicine against HIV/AIDS is created when you put yourself in charge of your medical care and make well-informed decisions about combining Western and Chinese treatments. Then you can create a treatment plan that provides the most effective therapy for your evolving physical and spiritual needs.

To help us on our tour of Western immunology, I have enlisted the help of two talented practitioners, Donald I. Abrams, M.D., a professor of clinical medicine at the University of San Francisco, assistant director of the AIDS Program at San Francisco General Hospital, and chairman of the Community Consortium, an AIDS research and advocacy group who has been working tirelessly since AIDS was first identified and was one of the first mainstream Western physicians open to studying the effects of alternative and Chinese medicine therapies; and Naomi Jay, R.N., Women's Health Practitioner and specialist in HIV-related research for men and women at the University of California's Departments of Stomatology and Adolescent Medicine.

THE BASICS OF THE IMMUNE SYSTEM

Western science has peered into the microscopic workings of the body and uncovered a marvelously complex and responsive network of cells, glands, and organs (including the spleen, thymus, lymph nodes, and bone marrow) that make up the body's immune system. With grace and speed they work together to coordinate the body's defense against attacks by harmful bacteria, viruses, fungi, cancer cells, and parasites.

The basic soldiers in the immune army are the phagocytes and lymphocytes (white blood cells). The most important phagocyte is the macrophage, produced in the bone marrow. It is the general housekeeper of the immune system, responsible for sweeping up and engulfing undesirables in the bloodstream. It holds the interlopers, or antigens, captive, and displays their unique insignias so that they are clearly identified as targets for destruction by other immune-system cells. The macrophage, when activated to attack a foreign body, also secretes a substance called interleukin-1, which activates a lymphocyte called a helper T (for thymus) cell, or a CD4+ cell. Interleukin-1 also stimulates a fever, which increases immune response.

The helper T cell binds to the macrophage and the engulfed antigen and begins to proliferate. Its offspring speed off to the lymph nodes and the spleen, where they stimulate production of killer T cells (also called CD8+ or suppressor T cells), the hit men of the immune system, and their partners, the B cells, the smart bombs that are responsible for producing the chemical, called an antibody, that attacks the offending antigen. The killer T cells also cause the body to secrete chemicals that can kill cells that may have already been infected.

Another essential component of the immune system includes the lymphoid organs: the bone marrow and the thymus. These organs produce and store the lymphocytes.

The bone marrow is where white and red blood cells and platelets are formed, as well as the macrophages and B cells.

The thymus is the organ in which T cells (such as the CD4+) mature.

The immune-system cells that are stored in these lymphoid organs migrate out into the body through both blood vessels and lymphatic vessels, which carry a fluid between the lymph nodes, which are clustered throughout the body. The immune cells that don't migrate into the bloodstream to track down enemy antigens gather within the lymph nodes to face the antigens as they circulate through.

Cellular and Humoral Immunity

This system of reacting to disease-causing trespassers is divided into two immune processes, *humoral immunity* and *cell-mediated immunity*. Humoral immunity is associated with the production by the B lymphocytes of antibodies that are precisely tailor-made to identify and vanquish specific antigens. (I consider this the Yin aspect of the immune system.) Cell-mediated immunity is associated with T cells that set out through the blood to track down and destroy an antigen. (I think this correlates closely with the concept of the Yang and Qi as essential forces in the battle against disease.)

Victory or Defeat

When the war between immune system and invader is won and an infection has been stopped from spreading, the body sends out so-called suppressor T cells (CD8+) to halt the action of the T cells and B cells.

But even the most highly tuned immune machine can't always win the battle against disease-spreading viruses, bacteria, fungi, and other infectious and destructive agents. In HIV disease the invading virus overwhelms the immune system's cells and produces illnesses, not only as a result of the presence of the virus, but by lowering overall resistance to disease and opening the body up to assault from infectious agents that would normally be destroyed by a healthy immune system.

THE WESTERN UNDERSTANDING OF HIV/AIDS

HIV is transmitted by intimate contact between contaminated fluids of an infected person and another person's mucous membrane or through direct contact with the blood. This occurs most easily when the infected person's viral load—the amount of HIV in the person's blood—is relatively high and the recipient's route of entry is large enough to let a sufficient amount of the virus into his or her bloodstream.

When the virus enters the body it seeks a host cell to attach to so it can borrow the additional biochemical components it needs to replicate its RNA. When it finds a host cell it likes, it attaches to receptors on that cell's outer wall, sends its RNA into the cell, and begins to make copies of itself, which migrate to other receptive cells and spread the infection. What makes HIV unusual is that it favors the immune system's own CD4+ cells.

As a result, the process of invasion and replication infects or destroys the very cells that the body uses to fight viral attacks. As more and more CD4+ cells are affected, they are less and less able to do their job in the immune system: The B cells are not summoned to fight the virus, but languish in the bone marrow; the killer T cells think they have nothing to do. And eventually, the chemical processes that go on inside an infected CD4+ cell damage uninfected CD4+ cells nearby: They begin to clump together, become immobilized, and eventually die. It is believed that although only a relatively few CD4+ cells are actually host to the invading HIV, vast numbers of them are killed off through the clumping process (also called syncytia).

In a healthy person there are about 1,000 to 1,500 CD4+ cells in a cubic millimeter of blood. As the virus kills off the body's CD4+ cells, the number begins to plummet, because so many more are being destroyed than the body can replace. But this happens gradually, over time.

STAGES OF HIV INFECTION AND PROGRESSION

The virus enters a person's bloodstream by hiding inside an infected cell that had been circulating in an infected person's blood and genital secretions. These fluids pass into another person through sexual contact, sharing needles,

THE CHARACTERISTICS OF HIV

HIV is a type of *retrovirus*—one that uses an enzyme called reverse transcriptase in its replication process. HIV has some distinct characteristics:

1. A tendency to infect the immune system's CD4+ cells and cells in the brain, central nervous system, and the skin, for example, which have the same HIV-friendly receptors that occur on the CD4+ cell.

2. HIV is particularly difficult for the immune system to control because initially it hides in healthy cells, particularly in the lymph nodes, instead of circulating in the blood.

3. The amount of circulating virus varies from person to person, making some individuals much more likely to be able to transmit the virus through their fluids than others. The highest levels of circulating virus are in people who are newly infected or who have advanced stages of AIDS. Transmission of HIV often occurs via HIV-infected cells circulating in the blood.

4. Genital secretions also are loaded with infected cells. During sexual contact these infected cells can be easily transmitted into the body if skin abrasions are present in the recipient's genital tract.

Adapted from *HIV and the Pathogenesis of AIDS* (American Society for Microbiology, 1994) by Jay A. Levy, M.D.

or blood transfusion. Once inside a new host, the virus begins replicating within the immune cells. During this phase of initial infection between 30 and 70 percent of people develop flulike symptoms: fever, nausea, aches, and pains. They may also develop oral ulcers, thrush (candidiasis in the mouth), and diarrhea. But these symptoms generally fade in a few days.

In addition, according to Eric Daar, M.D., assistant professor of medicine and director of AIDS research at Los Angeles' Cedars Sinai Medical Center, there are often biochemical changes that can only be detected in the laboratory: leukopenia (a decrease in the number of white blood cells), thrombocytopenia (a decrease in the number of blood platelets), and transaminases elevation (elevation in the levels of liver enzymes, indicating that there is liver stress). The passing of the flulike symptoms is a signal that the immune system is fighting back: The virus is being killed off by the T cells. In fact, according to Janice Giorgi, M.D., principal investigator of the Multicenter AIDS Cohort Study (MACS) Pathogenesis Research Laboratory, "If there were no immune defense against HIV, the entire immune system would be gone in about six weeks after infection." That only happens in cases of certain rare strains of the virus, or in people who are severely weakened by other chronic health problems.

Unfortunately, the initial efforts of the immune system do not eradicate the virus, but they usually hold the infection to a dull hum. It used to be thought that the virus was dormant while the HIV-positive person remained relatively healthy for months or years. That is now known to be untrue. During this time, the viral count may decline, but some infected cells are snared in the lymph nodes and HIV lurks there, replicating and infecting healthy immune cells as they circulate through the nodes. Over time, the lymph nodes break down, releasing the stored HIV into the blood, increasing viral load, and decreasing CD4+ counts.

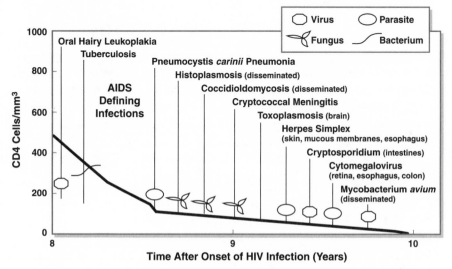

Figure 1. Major Opportunistic Infections in Advanced HIV Infection

There are some exceptions to this scenario: 6–8 percent of people who are HIV-positive are known as long-term nonprogressors. Some people contract HIV disease but have not gone on to have dramatically lowered CD4+ counts and high viral loads; others are able to resist serious opportunistic infection for years, despite unchanging but low CD4+ counts. These folks do offer some interesting insights into possible alternative approaches to treating HIV disease. In fact, the little research that there has been indicates the following possible factors in their longevity:

- The CD8+ cells (the killer T cells) in long-term survivors are three times more effective in suppressing the virus than in people with HIV who progress more rapidly from HIV infection to AIDS.
- Interleukin-2, a chemical, called a cytokine, that is known to be an important agent in controlling the virus's ability to replicate, is present in greater quantities and has enhanced activity in nonprogressors.[1]
- Overall, the viral load of long-term survivors has been found to be orders

of magnitude lower than that typically found in subjects with progressive disease.[2]

- Even in apparent nonprogressors when viral load is low, some researchers have found that viral replication does persist, however slowly.[3] Dr. C. Altisent, affiliated with the hospital Vall d'Hebron in Barcelona, Spain, reported in a letter in the *New England Journal of Medicine* that study results indicate that "HIV-1 infection progresses in a considerable percentage of long-term survivors, suggesting that long-term survivorship reflects a delay in the progression of the disease rather than the complete absence of progression."[4]

Other researchers have noted that long-term survivors seem to share certain personality traits, are often surrounded by loving support systems, and are altruistic themselves—working for the betterment of others who are ill. They are almost always committed to a lifestyle that includes a healthy diet, regular moderate exercise, avoiding drugs and excess stress, and responsible medical care. And many of them are not taking antiviral medication.

COUNTERACTING HIV'S PROGRESS

Western medicine currently has three main ways of treating HIV infection and associated disorders: (1) with antiretrovirals, (2) through immune restoration, and (3) through the use of preventive medications and strategies. I want to emphasize that because I am not a licensed Western medical doctor, I cannot prescribe Western drugs and I do not necessarily advocate their use; that is a decision for each person to make. What I do advocate is a carefully considered examination of the various opinions and latest studies so that you can make the best-informed choice. In the fast-changing world of HIV research, what we are certain today is the best treatment—like the three-drug cocktail and protease inhibitors—could be supplanted tomorrow by another medical breakthrough. In fact, we hope that is the case.

That said, let's look at current Western treatment.

Antiretroviral Drugs

As research continues into understanding how the virus colonizes other cells and how it replicates, it is becoming somewhat easier to create drugs that interfere with those processes. Some drugs, for example, protease inhibitors, prevent replication by denying the virus an essential chemical it needs to reproduce. But these antiretrovirals do not offer a "cure." What is needed are drugs that disable viruses lodged in all parts of the body—in the brain, the gut, the lymph nodes—and not just circulating in the bloodstream. Then an effective way to reverse the infection is conceivable in the future.

In the fall of 1997, *Science* published, "Identification of a Reservoir for

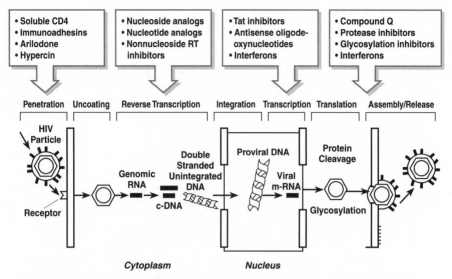

Figure 2. The Cellular Processes Impacted by Various Antiviral Medications
Antiviral medicines may prevent the replication of the HIV virus in several ways.
Some may keep the virus from entering potential host cells; others are designed
to interfere with enzyme actions that allow genetic replication, maturation of
new viruses, and their release into the bloodstream. For more details about
Figure 2 see Notes, Chapter 5, page 189.

HIV-1 in Patients of Highly Active Antiretroviral Therapy" (HAART) by Diana
Finzi and colleagues that confirmed what has long been suspected: That even
when using HAART—combining a protease inhibitor with nucleoside reverse
transcriptase inhibitors such as AZT and 3CT—the body retains resting or
latently infected CD4+ cells that are not detected in blood viral load tests. And
these cells can reawaken and begin replicating the virus anew.

In addition, there may be long-term negative results from aggressive and
early antiretroviral therapy: The immune system may be damaged, organ systems may suffer long-term injury, and the virus may become resistant to the
drugs and reemerge, resistant to other drug therapies.

In early 1997 the NIH convened the Panel to Define Principles of Therapy
in HIV Infection. They issued a finding that said, "Unless used correctly the
newest potent antiviral therapies will be of little clinical utility for treated
patients and may even compromise their ability to obtain long-term benefit
from other antiviral therapies." They made these basic recommendations:

1. All people with AIDS as defined by the Centers for Disease Control should
   receive combination antiretroviral therapy, preferably with three drugs,
   including a protease inhibitor.
2. The decisions about treatments for people with HIV/AIDS should be guided
   by regular monitoring of the amount of HIV in the patient's blood (viral

load) as well as the number of CD4+ T cells, the immune system cells that fight infection.

3. Treatment should begin with a three-drug cocktail and if treatment begins to fail, at least two of the drugs should be changed. Treatment with only two drugs in general is considered less than optimal and treatment with only one drug is not recommended. (The use of AZT alone as a preventive measure against transmission of HIV to a fetus is recommended.)

In the meantime, the new and increasingly sophisticated blood viral load tests are very useful. Newly infected people can obtain a diagnosis quite soon after transmission and, whether or not they choose to use antiviral drugs, can take steps to act quickly and aggressively to protect others from infection with HIV and to protect themselves from progressing toward development of more serious disease. (The only diagnostic tests previously available were the Western Blot and ELISA, which look for the presence of antibodies to HIV and the P24 antigen test. The first two generally give an accurate positive reading from four weeks to six months after infection and the P24 is not able to detect the presence of this HIV-related marker in all infected individuals. The viral load test can detect the presence of HIV RNA almost immediately.)

Immune Restoration

A second, and increasingly popular, method of treating HIV infection is immune restoration—that is, reversing the damage that HIV does to the immune system so the body can successfully fight, and vanquish, HIV and opportunistic infections.

In many ways I feel this is where East and West come closest: Chinese medicine is based on the premise that the role of a practitioner is to help the body heal itself. Immune restoration is focused on precisely the same goal.

Challenges Facing Immune Restoration

Replacing damaged and destroyed immune cells in a manner that allows them to be fully functional is a complex process. Scientists are only now beginning to understand what is required to make an immune-compromised system fully functional again. The following are some of the most recent innovations that may help the HIV-compromised immune system reclaim its disease-fighting powers.

Protease inhibitors. The new three-drug cocktails, which include a protease inhibitor, can reduce viral loads to nearly undetectable levels. Scientists conjecture that that may allow the immune system to rebound, replacing damaged and destroyed T cells.

Interleukin-2. IL-2 is a body chemical that stimulates the immune system to produce more T cells. Recent studies indicate that a wide range of people with

CD4+ counts may be helped by IL-2 therapy if it is used in conjunction with antiviral therapy capable of reducing the viral load to insignificant levels.

T cell culture and reintroduction. Increasing the number of immune cells—particularly CD4+ and CD8+—can also be accomplished by removing some uninfected ones from a person with HIV and nurturing the cells in a laboratory. When they have multiplied many times over, they are reintroduced into the infected person, giving the immune system a jump start.

There are obstacles to these methods of restoring immune system cells however: The triple-drug cocktail and IL-2 may encourage the T cells that remain in the body to multiply, but HIV often eradicates specialized subgroups of immune cells from the body and when they are gone, helping existent immune cells multiply will not regrow these missing varieties or reintroduce their unique disease-fighting functions.

For example, some people who take IL-2 experience a dramatic rise in their CD4+ counts, bringing them up to levels that should eliminate the risk for opportunistic infections such as cytomegalovirus (CMV). Yet they still contract the disease. Why? The T cells that were programmed to fight off CMV have all been destroyed by the HIV infection. IL-2 cannot restore those cells, nor can it stimulate the body to produce fresh ones that can be programmed to fight CMV anew (at least not in people with advanced AIDS). So despite a high CD4+ count, these HIV-positive people are not able to resist the virus when they are exposed to it.

Another possible drawback to these therapies for those with high viral loads: The new T cells simply provide a larger target for the circulating HIV and they become infected before they can provide benefits.

Blocking HIV's action. HIV invades the body's immune cells by docking on the outside of the cells on small protrusions called receptors. These sites give HIV places to attach to the healthy cells so they can then enter and replicate within them. Keeping the virus from getting a foothold on the immune cells would seem to make it impossible for the virus to replicate. Research indicates people who appear to be resistant to HIV (and there are some) are missing a receptor known as CCR5. Genetic manipulation may one day allow these HIV-resistant cells to provide immunity to the greater population.

Thymus transplants. While the methods mentioned above are potentially helpful, another way to fight HIV may be to restore the body's ability to create what are called naive immune cells. These brand-new cells, not yet marked for specific disease-fighting functions, can go out into the bloodstream and battle newly encountered diseases.

Such cells begin life in the bone marrow, and the T cells among them then migrate to the thymus gland for maturation. Unfortunately, the thymus gland often is damaged severely in the course of HIV infection and its ability to mature new T cells may diminish dramatically. That's why research is focused on ways to transplant healthy thymus tissue into the body—even small pieces of the gland inserted into the thoracic cavity may be sufficient to generate naive T cells.

These are but a few of the more interesting approaches currently under investigation. This is a field that changes rapidly and the best way to find out about emerging developments is to stay in touch with Project Inform's Immune Restoration Project.[5] (See Appendix 6, page 218.) This project provides bulletins and updates and holds a highly respected annual think tank on these issues.

Preventive Therapies: Countering Opportunistic Infections

The third way Western medicine treats HIV disease and related disorders is through preventive therapy of opportunistic infections. There are medications that may prevent even those with very low CD4+ counts from contracting PCP (*Pneumocystis carinii* pneumonia), MAC (*Mycobacterium avium* complex), and possibly CMV (cytomegalovirus), and some fungal infections.

CORRELATING CHINESE AND WESTERN CONCEPTS

There are many similarities in the way Chinese and Western medicine view the impact of HIV on the body's systems. Here's a brief look at some of the correlations.

• *The lymph system and the Spleen System.* Western medicine focuses on the role of the lymphatic system—including the spleen, thymus, lymph nodes, bone marrow, and some mucous membranes, particularly in the gut, genital tract, mouth, and nose—as an important component of the immune system and a target for HIV.

In Chinese medicine, the Spleen Organ System fulfills functions that are remarkably similar to the various organs, glands, and tissues in the lymph system. It provides protection from disease and keeps the blood healthy and the inner workings of the body, particularly digestion, operating harmoniously. When HIV attacks the body, it affects the Spleen System, particularly the gut. And when the Spleen System becomes severely depleted it triggers disharmonies in related systems such as the Lung System, and that triggers disharmonies in the mouth and nose and lungs.

• *The lymph system and the Jin-Ye.* The lymph nodes are like filters along the lymphatic channels, which carry the lymphatic fluid. When the lymphatic system becomes overwhelmed with HIV and the immune system weakens, the lymph nodes wither. The lymphatic fluid, so vital to making sure that immune-system cells are available throughout the body as needed, functions much like the Jin-Ye, which travels through the channels and supports the very essence of health and well-being.

• *The blood and the Xue.* Lymph nodes have a rich blood supply and this is related to the Spleen System's role in bringing nutrient energy to the Xue (blood), as well as the role of the blood in transporting infected T cells to the spleen and other lymph tissues.

The bone marrow is another important part of the lymphatic system and is essential for production of blood. Millions of lymphocytes are scattered throughout the bone marrow, making it a prime target for HIV. In Chinese medicine, Xue (blood) production is directly controlled by the Spleen, yet the bone marrow—which plays a fundamental part in blood production—is associated with the Kidney. This accounts for the development of Kidney disharmonies as HIV infection moves more deeply into the body.

• *The thymus and the Jing.* The thymus is where T cells mature from undifferentiated lymphocytes. This correlates with the manner in which Jing (the parent of the immature T cell) and Qi (the force that allows the T cell to mature) create a strong systemic defense against disharmony.

• *The gastrointestinal system and the Spleen and Stomach Systems.* HIV infection infects the mucous membrane of the gastrointestinal tissue. In Chinese medicine, as we've seen, the Spleen and the Stomach are associated with digestion, and treatments directed at restoring harmony to the Spleen and Stomach Systems can be effective against HIV-related gastrointestinal disorders.

HIV-RELATED WESTERN DIAGNOSES AND ASSOCIATED TRADITIONAL CHINESE MEDICINE (TCM) PATTERNS OF DISHARMONY

Western Diagnosis	Selected Possible TCM Patterns
Antiretroviral syndrome (acute HIV infection)	Toxic Heat Excess Heat Heat in the Xue
Pneumocystis carinii pneumonia	Qi Deficiency Yin Deficiency Lung Heat Lung Damp Heat
Shingles *(Herpes zoster)*	Heat in the channels Damp Heat in the channels Toxic Heat
Neuropathy	Dampness in the channels Qi and Xue Deficiency Xue Stagnation Cold Stagnation

Western Diagnosis	Selected Possible TCM Patterns
Diarrhea	Spleen Qi Deficiency
	Spleen Yang Deficiency
	Spleen Damp Heat
	Damp Heat in the Large Intestine
MAC (*Mycobacterium avium* complex)	Yin Deficiency
	Xue Deficiency
	Toxic Heat
Dementia	Shen disturbance
	Lack of Shen
Depression	Liver Qi Stagnation
	Shen disturbance
	Heart Xue Deficiency
Anxiety	Heart Fire
	Liver Fire
Candidiasis	Spleen Dampness
	Spleen Damp Heat
	Liver Qi Stagnation
Wasting disease	Spleen Qi Deficiency
(cytomegalovirus)	Spleen Yang Deficiency
	Spleen Yin Deficiency
CMV retinitis	Kidney Deficiency
Hepatitis	Liver/Gallbladder Damp Heat
	Spleen Damp Cold
	Spleen Damp Heat
	Spleen Deficiency
	Qi Stagnation
	Qi Deficiency
	Xue Deficiency
	Xue Stagnation
Cervical dysplasia	Toxic Heat with:
	Yin Deficiency in Kidney and Liver
	Damp Heat in Liver channel

Western Diagnosis	**Selected Possible TCM Patterns**
Kaposi's sarcoma	Xue Stagnation with:
	Spleen Qi Deficiency
	Kidney Qi Deficiency
Toxoplasmosis	Lack of Shen
	Liver Yang rising
	Toxic Heat

PART III

Restoring Balance to the Mind/Body/Spirit:

The Basic Chicken Soup Chinese Medicine Clinic Program for Managing Early HIV Infection

Chinese medicine offers those who are HIV-positive a powerful means for maintaining physical and emotional strength and counteracting the development of opportunistic infections.

The four pillars of therapy are nutritional modification, herbs, acupuncture and moxibustion, and Qi Gong exercise and meditation. And although Chinese medicine is highly individualized (that's what makes it so hard to study in double-blind controlled environments), I have developed a basic regime using these four therapies that is beneficial to most people who are HIV-positive.

This Basic HIV+ Program follows a protocol, or plan, developed and refined through 15 years of clinical experience with thousands of HIV-positive people at Quan Yin Acupuncture and Herb Center, and at the nonprofit Quan Yin Healing Arts Center, where I am founder and director of education and research, and at my private treatment facility, Chicken Soup Chinese Medicine, all in San Francisco.

So let's take a look at the dietary, herbal, acupuncture, and Qi Gong therapies that we recommend for immune-related deficiencies, disharmonies, and diseases. Treatment protocols for particular HIV-associated syndromes and diseases appear in Part IV.

6

Nurturing the
Mind/Body/Spirit:
The HIV+ Dietary Programs

My diet had always been about 75 percent junk food, even when I
was in medical school. In fact, it took me nine years after I was
diagnosed before I realized that I needed to take advantage of the
power of food to help make me stronger and finally hooked up
with a nutritionist. But it wasn't easy to change my eating habits;
anyone who's tried will tell you that you have to take it slow, and
reeducate yourself and your taste buds.

—Wayne B., M.D., diagnosed in 1984

Chicken Soup's three-part dietary therapy program provides your first
line of defense against the most powerful cause of chronic debilitation associated with HIV infection: wasting. It combines an aggressive approach to managing what you eat with nutritional supplementation and Western medicines,
when needed, to build lean-muscle mass and stop weight loss.

"We know now that a person's nutritional status changes very shortly after
initial infection," says Mary Romeyn, M.D., an internist at San Francisco's
Saint Francis Memorial Hospital and author of *Nutrition and HIV: A New Model
for Treatment,* second edition (Jossey-Bass, 1998). "In a sense, wasting begins
to be a problem from the first and everything a person does to treat the
disease and take care of themselves should be designed to prevent weight loss
and maintain lean-muscle mass."

I can't emphasize enough how important it is to weigh yourself weekly and
to have your lean-muscle mass evaluated at least three times a year by a
person trained to do so, even if you don't appear to be getting thinner. Wasting and nutritional deficiencies are a problem even among those who appear
healthy. And nutritional support needs to be provided from diagnosis on.

If possible, don't wait until you begin noticeably losing weight to take
preventive steps. However, it's never too late to take positive action to halt
weight loss. If you are currently losing weight, you should immediately increase your food intake and go for diagnostic screening to make sure you

aren't suffering from an undiagnosed—and treatable—opportunistic infection such as parasites, MAC (*Mycobacterium avium* complex), candidiasis, or lymphoma. Then you can establish a program for weight gain that is tailored to your constitutional needs.

The current definition of HIV wasting syndrome is loss of 10 percent of body weight in three months' time and chronic diarrhea or fevers, in the absence of any disease other than the primary HIV infection. This is often accompanied by CD4+ counts below 100 per milliliter of blood, although studies suggest that malnutrition is independent of CD4+ counts and offers another strongly predictive assessment of disease outcome.[1] That's why prompt action to halt wasting is imperative: Regardless of what infection or syndrome a person appears to die from, it is the reduction in lean-muscle body mass— what Dr. Romeyn calls "a special and complex type of starvation"—that appears to determine longevity.[2]

Several useful tests can be run to monitor your nutritional levels that will help your Chinese practitioner and your Western doctor provide the support you need. According to Dr. Romeyn, the most important blood test is for albumin, a substance produced by the liver. She recommends that you check every three months to track developing metabolic problems: Readings below 3.0 grams per deciliter (one tenth of a liter) of blood demand aggressive intervention and she says she begins to worry at levels of 3.7 or lower. A test for total iron binding capacity (TIBC) is also useful because it shows protein wasting sooner than the albumin test. Lastly, the Prealbumin test provides more targeted information than the TIBC, but it can take four days to get results, and in a situation that calls for immediate action that is too long to wait.

See Dr. Romeyn's book (Appendix 5) for details on these tests.

WESTERN MANAGEMENT OF METABOLIC DYSFUNCTIONS

The Western solutions to wasting include treatments that inhibit abnormal absorption and limit inflammation, and anabolic agents that stimulate the creation of lean-muscle mass.

Several therapies have been tested with indication of positive results.

- Anabolic steroids such as oxandrolone have been shown to increase protein metabolism and reduce protein breakdown (catabolism)—in fact, according to Donald Kottler, M.D., of St. Luke's–Roosevelt Hospital in New York City, who is a specialist in issues of HIV-related weight loss, 93 percent of study participants in an uncontrolled study who were given anabolic steroids gained weight.
- There is also evidence that daily shots of synthetic recombinant growth hormone (somatotropin) lead to added lean-muscle mass and often work

when other therapies fail.[3] Unfortunately, this treatment costs around $50,000 a year.

- Appetite stimulants such as megestrol acetate have been found to add fat and fluid weight, but unfortunately not lean muscle.
- Dronabinol, an antinausea appetite stimulant made from a chemical similar to the active ingredient in marijuana, often makes the user feel too loopy.
- Testosterone enanthate, the male sex hormone, can be used to add muscle bulk in both men and women. Initial studies are promising and the drug is relatively inexpensive. Nandrolone, an anabolic steroid, is sometimes used with testosterone.
- Thalidomide appears to be helpful to some people by blocking production of tumor necrosis factor, which is implicated in wasting.
- In extreme cases, usually in the later stages of AIDS, total parenteral nutrition (TPN)—the intravenous infusion of nutrients—may be needed. The cost is often prohibitive, however, and it is used to prevent starvation rather than to build muscle mass.

CHINESE MEDICINE'S UNDERSTANDING OF WASTING

When a person is HIV-positive, Toxic Heat assaults the Spleen and Stomach Systems, the very core of the body's food-processing engine, where Qi is extracted from food and strong Xue (blood) is created.

From the initial infection with HIV the Spleen and Stomach are distressed, and that begins a cascade of disharmonies in Essential Substances and associated Organ Systems. These contribute to the development of one or both types of wasting associated with HIV infection: primary weight loss and wasting associated with metabolic disharmonies.

Primary Weight Loss

This is triggered by Toxic Heat and the resulting inflammation in the gut and disruption in the Spleen and the Stomach. Those who are losing weight due to Toxic Heat can regain weight—including lean-muscle mass—through increased intake of calories and protein, control of diarrhea, exercise, and therapy to increase absorption in the gut and stimulate appetite.

Sometimes, however, primary weight loss may happen because of other factors surrounding the assault of Toxic Heat and infection with HIV, and that calls for additional remedies.

Negative Reaction to Medication

Western therapy: Evaluate and weigh risk/benefits before making decision about discontinuing medication.

Chinese therapy: Design herbal formulas and acupuncture routines to help alleviate negative side effects of Western medication. These are highly effective. See individual treatment programs in Part IV for more details.

Presence of Undiagnosed Opportunistic Infection

Western therapy: Thorough ongoing diagnostic attention from doctor.

Chinese therapy: Thorough ongoing diagnostic attention from practitioner.

Lack of Access to High-Nutrition Meals

Western therapy: Use shortcuts to get nutrients, such as rice or soy-based weight-gain drinks. Drink them at room temperature or warm, not refrigerated.

Eastern therapy: A Japanese fermented rice drink, amazake, is sweet and calorie-laden. Drink it at room temperature or warmed up.

Depression

Western therapy: Antidepressants.

Chinese therapy: Reharmonize the Shen using a combination of diet, acupuncture, meditation, exercise, and herbs.

HIV-Related Gastroparesis

This is vomiting and nausea caused by the inability of the stomach to empty correctly.

Western therapy: Metoclopramide or cisapride.

Chinese therapy: Herbs, diet, and acupuncture to correct Food Stagnation in the Stomach and to harmonize Spleen and Stomach Systems.

Loss of Appetite

Western therapy: Megestrol acetate or dronabinol.

Chinese therapy: Acupuncture, sweet-tasting foods, Chinese Curing Pills (also called Pill Curing), which are available at many health food stores, and herbal formulas prescribed by your practitioner.

Mouth Pain Caused by Gum and Dental Problems

Western therapy: Dental care as needed.
Chinese therapy: Herbal mouthwash and acupuncture.

Wasting Associated with Metabolic Disharmonies

This second type of weight loss, triggered by deeper changes in the body's metabolism, is associated with deficient Qi and Xue, and especially severe Spleen Deficiency (muscle mass is associated with the Spleen in Chinese medicine) that set in when Toxic Heat moves deeper into the body. It corresponds to the Western concept of the HIV-wasting syndrome that is due to metabolic imbalances.

Researchers have discovered that the metabolic changes associated with HIV wasting produce very different bodily responses than does simple starvation: HIV-related wasting causes much greater loss of lean-muscle mass in relation to the amount of fat lost than does a starvation disorder such as anorexia nervosa. What this means in everyday terms is that when you are HIV-positive you are burning up protein and lean-muscle mass to feed your hungry body instead of fat stores, as is usual when the body senses that it is being deprived of needed food and nutrients. Another metabolic difference between HIV-associated wasting and simple starvation, according to Marc Hellerstein, M.D., Ph.D., an assistant professor of medicine at the University of California–San Francisco and a specialist in the metabolic changes underlying HIV wasting, is that the liver's conversion of body protein into glucose and glucose into fat triggers a *rise* in triglyceride levels—the exact opposite of what usually happens in starvation. And he points out that metabolic disturbances often cause HIV-infected people who gain weight through various remedies to put on fat and fluids, not lean-muscle mass, as might be expected in normal weight gain. Another interesting distinction, according to Dr. Kottler, is that while standard starvation causes the body to slow down so that resting energy expenditure falls to conserve calories, in HIV-related wasting the resting energy expenditure seems to actually increase—in some cases as much as 29 percent—making it harder and harder to consume enough calories to stave off weight loss.[4] This is characteristic of Spleen Yin Deficiency.

PROMOTING DIGESTIVE HEALTH

No matter what has triggered your weight loss, it is vital that digestion and absorption be improved. Both are hampered by the presence of HIV itself, associated infections and syndromes, medications, and the various biochemical problems that result from the progressive cascade of Organ System disharmonies. According to Lark Lands, M.S., Ph.D., a health educator who has spent the past nine years developing information on a "total aggressive approach to AIDS" and who is very concerned with the impact of diet and nutritional supplements, HIV depletes supplies of hydrochloric acid in the stomach; tablets to replenish it, such as Solgar Beta-Pepsin, may help. She cautions against overdoing it, however, and advises people who are HIV-positive to start with small doses, building up to the level needed. Alternatives to the pills include Chinese green tea and plant bitters that stimulate the production of stomach acid. In addition, there are Chinese Curing Pills and other herbal formulas.

Chinese Dietary Therapy Basics

Chinese medicine recognizes that food has an impact on the mind/body/spirit in many ways. If you open yourself up to the basic principles, you can nurture your sensitivity to the power of food and start to harness its curing effects.

Eating Qi

Gu (Grain) Qi enters the body through food and joins with Kong (Air) Qi, which enters your body through breathing, and Yuan (Prenatal) Qi, which you receive from your parents. Together these form Zheng (Normal) Qi (what we mean when we simply say Qi), which gives motion and power to the body. A healthy supply of Normal Qi allows you to gain strength from stored Ying (Nutritive) Qi in the food you eat. When the Spleen and Stomach are attacked by Toxic Heat and digestions become impaired, the body may lack sufficient supplies of Grain Qi, leading to more severe Qi Deficiency and further Organ System complications.

A Spirit Sandwich

Your diet also shapes your Shen, the Essential Substance that creates the spirit and makes each of us uniquely human. Shen can be depleted when the diet is unbalanced or if disharmony in the other Essential Substances and Organ Systems makes it difficult for the body to absorb the nutrition from food. In the management of HIV disease and in maintaining maximum immune strength, a positive attitude is essential. In addition, depression can lead to lack of appetite and further wasting. Protecting your Shen through careful diet, meditation, and supportive acupuncture contributes to your overall health in many ways.

Essence Soup

Jing, the Essential Substance that is the very essence of life, is inextricably intertwined with Qi. Without a constant supply of fresh Jing from the food we eat, the stresses of life would consume the Jing we are born with and we would wither and die prematurely.

The Energetics of Food

In Chinese medicine philosophy, food not only acts as a building block for Essential Substances and Organ Systems but can also, in and of itself, create disharmony in the mind/body/spirit or help restore balance to distressed bodily systems. A healthful diet uses these Energetics to achieve balance and harmony. The Energetics are able to cool or warm the metabolism and Organ Systems, moisturize or dry the Organ Systems, and increase or decrease the flow of Qi, Jing, and Xue.

When you take in a balance of energetics, the Essential Substances and Organ Systems thrive, but if your diet contains too much or too little of the energetics then you may develop a disharmony: They may be overwhelmed by excess dryness or moisture; or too much coolness or heat. These imbalances can trigger excesses or deficiencies in Qi, Jing, or Xue (blood) and disharmony in the Shen (spirit).

How to Keep Energetics Well Balanced in Your Diet

- Eat mostly warm foods, which sustain the digestive system.
- Eliminate raw foods almost totally from your diet. In Chinese medicine, raw food is understood to be depleting, since your body must expend energy to warm it up to body temperature so it can be digested. This can be particularly exhausting for those with chronic immune and viral disorders. In fact, the Chinese call the mixture in the stomach the 100-Degree Soup.
- Chew your food well to cherish the available supply of Protective Qi. This takes a burden off the digestive system and helps reserve the digestive fires that help the Spleen and Stomach Systems to digest and disperse food's powerful components. Since the Spleen and Stomach Systems are already weakened in those who are HIV-positive, you want to protect the Organ Systems and help them stay as strong as possible.
- Avoid drinking a lot of liquids while or immediately after eating. They dampen the digestive fires.
- Eliminate frozen and iced foods from your diet completely. Again, they put a strain on the already taxed Stomach and Spleen Systems.
- Try to eat only pesticide- and hormone-free foods. You don't need any additional strain on your system from unknown chemical assailants.
- A non-Chinese imperative: Drink only filtered water, to eliminate bacterial contaminants that are particularly dangerous for those with immune-compromised systems. The best filters are ones that use reverse osmosis to extract pollutants and chemical additives. They are far more effective than carbon filters and are much less expensive than a bulky water distillation system. For details on obtaining filters, see Appendix 8.
- Another non-Chinese imperative: Wash all fruits and vegetables in a

dilute Clorox solution to eliminate the chance of some opportunistic bacterial infections.

The Power of Food Flavors

Chinese medicine also recognizes that each of the five basic flavors of foods—sour, bitter, sweet, spicy, and salt—affects the harmony or disharmony of the mind/body/spirit. Each food may have a flavor that is cold or cool, hot or warm: For example, tofu is sweet and cool; chicken is sweet and warm. A balanced diet is composed of mostly sweet, warm foods; cold, spicy, bitter, salty, and sour are best eaten as accents. As a general rule: A little of any flavor tonifies. *Tonify* is a common Chinese medicine term that is used to mean "strengthen and support." A salty flavor concentrates. Sour contracts. Bitter descends. Sweet expands and spicy disperses. No flavors are bad except when taken in excess or when a disharmony is present.

One thing to remember is that sweet taste stimulates appetite (and tonifies the Stomach and Spleen) while you're eating, and that makes natural sweets such as cooked fruits and some vegetables good foods for those who have lost their interest in eating or find they can't taste well (which happens frequently as a result of HIV infection and various medications). So include a sweet food in each meal, to help keep your appetite healthy.

You Are Also *How* You Eat

Taking nutrition into your body is not a mechanical or biochemical process that can be satisfactorily achieved without thought to your attitude and environment. The therapeutic power of food stems in part from how you cook, serve, and consume it.

Chinese medicine recommends that you take the time to honor your food, and yourself, while eating. Enjoy the flavors, textures, and smells of the food while you prepare it. And then find a quiet place to eat it, where you can concentrate on receiving the nurturing gift that it brings to your body.

This may all sound like so much hooey, but if for just one week you turn off the TV, don't eat at your desk or in the car, and make mealtime a healing event, you—and your digestive system—will feel much healthier. You will also find that you automatically make healthier food choices because you are actually tasting the food and tuning in to how it makes you feel. Just watch your cat or dog eat—they are completely focused on tasting every single bite of food.

THE BASIC DIETARY THERAPY PROGRAM

Never start any program without consulting with your doctors and practitioners, nor if you are in the throes of an acute illness. And don't continue any program if you find that your weight loss continues or that you are becoming more nauseated or are experiencing increased diarrhea.

This program has two components, the daily journal and the five-phase cleansing diet.

You should keep a journal for two weeks when you first begin your dietary program. You tune in to and keep a record of exactly what you eat, when you eat it, and how it makes you feel. Then you'll be ready to start on whatever aspect of the program suits you and your current level of vitality and health. You then revisit the journal every three months for a week, tracking your eating habits to compare changes in types and quantities of food you are eating and to see if you have developed any new sensitivities over time. This allows you to adjust your diet to make sure you are getting sufficient calories and protein and to avoid foods that are currently upsetting your digestion.

DAILY JOURNAL

For one to two weeks before going to visit your Chinese practitioner, keep a daily journal. In it record the following:

- Everything you eat and drink, noting the time of day.
- Any bodily symptoms such as headaches, gas pains, fatigue, blood sugar swings, stiff neck, and the time of day they appear.
- Your physical activities—walking, climbing stairs, working out, dancing, sitting at a desk, watching TV, naps, and for how long you do them.
- Your nighttime sleep patterns.
- Your digestion and patterns of elimination. Of particular importance are the times you are hungry, bloated, gassy, or constipated or have loose stools, acid indigestion, etc. Also note how often you urinate and what color the urine is.
- Your emotions; be specific about when certain feelings arise and their causes, if you can identify them.
- Your intake of prescription drugs, recreational drugs, alcohol, and cigarettes/cigars/chewing tobacco.
- Your mental clarity—when you feel groggy, sharp-witted, or experience fuzzy thinking.

Don't try to correlate the symptoms and activities and the food you eat—at least not yet. Simply take note. Later, as you look back over the record, you will see whether any patterns are evident. For example, on days you eat chicken, do you always develop a rash, or the day after you have salad, do you feel chilled? You and your practitioner will look over the record together and work out dietary and lifestyle adjustments for you to try.

THE FIVE-PHASE CLEANSING DIET

This program is designed to identify food-related disharmonies, to eliminate stress on the digestive system, and to give the body a rest from potentially antagonistic foods. Remember, Chinese medicine is about moderation, and you don't want to exacerbate a deficiency that already exists. So if your CD4+ count is below 500, your viral load is above 3,000, or you are losing weight or suffer from chronic diarrhea, skip the first three phases of the cleansing diet and simply follow the guidelines in the fourth and fifth phases. Remember also that this plan should always be done under the supervision of a licensed practitioner who is knowledgeable about your overall health and understands your condition in terms of Chinese and Western diagnosis and evaluation.

If you do go through the cleansing diet, your goals are to follow the basic Chinese medicine guidelines for healthful eating and to construct a daily diet you can stick to, using the foods that make you feel the strongest.

In this regime, you may follow each step for anywhere from a day to a week, depending on your current condition and how the step makes you feel.

Please do not use any step that may cause weight loss if you are already losing weight. Do not continue with any step that causes too much weakness or weight loss. There is no absolute right or wrong—remember, this should make you feel better, not cause stress, starvation, or increase your depletion.

In Phases 2–4, you may use a rice-based protein powder or predigested protein as a supplement if necessary to prevent weakness and weight loss. Avoid milk-based protein powder, which may cause diarrhea. Some people find that soy creates the same problem.

When you have completed the cleansing diet, you should have more normal bowel function and improved absorption and utilization of food.

Phase 1: Tonifying the Spleen and Stomach
Duration: one to seven days.

Foods for Phase 1
Limit diet to the following foods and pure water. You may do this for a day—or even part of a day—if that is best for your current constitutional needs. Remember: Do not do anything that causes you to lose significant weight. For those who are already experiencing wasting this is particularly important.

• *Miso broth.* Miso, or fermented soy and grain paste, contains friendly bacteria that replenish important intestinal flora that aid digestion. We recommend Mugi (barley) miso with some Mellow Yellow (light yellow miso) in warm weather; use Hatcho (dark) miso only when it is very cold.

• *Brown rice cereal.* Available at health food stores.

• *Vegetable broth and juice from carrots, celery, daikons, watercress, or beets.* Room-temperature or warm vegetable juices are considered generally okay in

---

TO MAKE A VEGETABLE MISO SOUP

Ingredients
1 cup kombu, hijiki, or other sea vegetable
1 cup chard, kale, or other dark greens
1/2 cup sliced carrots
5 teaspoons miso
5 cups filtered water

1. Rinse sea vegetables in cold water for 10 minutes; wipe dry to remove excess salt. Dice.

2. Wash and dice other vegetables and set aside.

3. Place sea vegetables in saucepan with 5 cups filtered water and boil for 10 minutes. Turn off heat. Do not drain.

4. Mix 5 teaspoons miso with 1/4 cup of the water in which you cooked the sea vegetables.

5. When well mixed, stir into saucepan with the sea vegetables and water.

6. Add remaining vegetables and cook on low simmer until done. Do not boil water once miso is added or you will kill the healthful bacteria.

---

small quantities because the body does not have to make such an effort to "cook" and digest them as it does if the vegetables are raw and eaten whole. You may also heat the vegetable juices and broths for souplike servings. Lentil broth (cook lentils, strain off the water, and drink as a soup) may also be used in addition to the vegetable broths. And unsalted pure vegetable powder such as Jensen's Broth can be added to broths and juices to boost nutritional impact and flavor.

Remember to rinse all veggies in a dilute solution of Clorox, one half teaspoon per quart of water, for ten minutes and to rinse off solution well before eating or juicing. Use filtered water. And avoid all raw fruit and vegetables in restaurants or if not properly prepared.

Further Points

• Eliminate caffeine, alcohol, sugar, and foods to which you know you are allergic.

• Drink only filtered water to avoid cryptosporidia (which can cause chronic diarrhea) and other parasites and bacterial contaminants. Carry water with you during the day and avoid all ice from unfiltered water. Removing cryptosporidia from water requires a filter that removes particles smaller than 2 microns (less than one ten-thousandth of an inch). If that's not available boil all tap water for at least five minutes to make it safe for drinking.

Bottled water is another option; according to the organization Gay Men's

Health Crisis (GMHC), some bottled water is filtered well enough to trap cryptosporidia. The following companies report that they use safe filters: Deer Park, Great Bear, Naya, and Poland Springs. Check with the water companies in your area for information.

Home water systems that claim to remove cryptosporidia include Multi-Pure Drinking Water Systems, whose models are tested and certified by the EPA and the National Sanitation Foundation; and Neolife Water Dome, which removes particles less than .4 microns in size and larger.

Phase 2: Building the Xue

Duration: one to seven days. You may skip and go directly to Phase 3 if you wish, should you need to increase food intake to maintain weight.

Foods for Phase 2

Add steamed fresh organic root and green, leafy vegetables such as carrots, turnips, kohlrabi, parsnips, yams, burdock, beets, broccoli, kale, and chard to the Phase 1 foods.

Phase 3: Balancing the Kidney and Cooling the Internal Heat

Duration: one to seven days. You may skip to Phase 4 or 5 if you need to do so to maintain strength and weight.

Foods for Phase 3

Add cooked, organic grains such as brown rice and barley to foods above. If you have diarrhea, add unbleached white rice or white basmati rice. Do not eat wheat, corn, oats, or any bread products.

Phase 4: The Balanced Spleen and Stomach

Duration: one to seven days.

You may simply adopt the guidelines in this phase without going through the previous cleansing steps if you need to eat a fuller diet every day. The balanced nutrition outlined in this phase offers the low-fat, high-protein, calorie-intense diet you need to maintain weight, while protecting your digestive system from unnecessary irritants.

Foods for Phase 4

At this point you should expand your diet every day to include a wider variety of organic products and meat and fish. But don't overwhelm your system with "new" foods. Then, as you add foods back into your diet you can make special note of any symptoms that might arise—gas, bloating, skin irritations, stuffy nose, or sinus congestion, for example. If you think you see a correlation, eliminate the offending food from your diet—but make sure you adjust your other foods so you maintain necessary nutrition. Your best bet is to remain lactose-free by eliminating dairy products from your diet, since people with HIV infection tend to be more lactose-intolerant.

Phase 5: Your Life-Diet

Foods for Phase 5

Once you go through Phase 4 and have added a variety of foods to your diet that seem to sit well with you, and your digestion is regular and complete, you will have entered Phase 5: Now your digestive system has rested. You have tuned in to foods that make you feel strong and have identified those that may trigger digestive distress. Using this information, move on to the antiwasting diet so that you are able to resist weight loss as effectively as possible.

F.Y.I.

For more information on wasting and other health issues related to HIV infection, you can order back copies of the May 1995 issue of *Treatment Issues* from GMHC for $3. For a complete set of back issues send $25 to GMHC, Treatment Education, 129 West 20th St., New York, NY 10011. The suggested donation for a subscription is $35/year (11 issues) for individuals. Information is also available through PWA Health Group, 212-255-0520, and *BETA, Bulletin for Experimental Treatment for AIDS,* published by the San Francisco AIDS Foundation. See Appendix 5 for address.

THE ANTIWASTING DIET

The Antiwasting Diet is the general diet to follow every day. It contains a comprehensive program of nutritional support including recipes and nutritional guidelines, exercises to build lean-muscle mass, herbs and acupuncture to promote absorption of nutrients, and techniques to help you retain your appetite and sense of taste. This diet is valuable for everyone who is HIV-positive, including those who are taking protease inhibitors and the three-drug cocktails. Although you will gain weight and appear to reverse wasting with these medications, data presented at an NIH conference in the spring of 1996 showed that Highly Active Antiretroviral Therapy—HAART—was adding fluid and fat, not lean-muscle mass.

NUTRITIONAL GUIDELINES

Fluids

Water is essential to keep the digestive system working and helps create Jin-Ye, the bodily fluids that lubricate the Stomach and Spleen. Again, all water should be filtered and free of bacterial contamination. Use a filter that removes contaminants of 2 microns or smaller. Carry water with you through the day and avoid ice unless it is made from filtered water. Cryptosporidium can be acquired at any T cell count. Remember: Don't drink too much fluid during or after eating; it puts out the digestive fires.

Other fluids such as vegetable broths or juices, high-protein drinks, and liquid nutritional supplements can provide power-packed extra calories and protein to supplement what you eat.

> To help determine your optimum nutritional levels of calories, protein, and other nutrients, you may want to consult with a registered dietitian or nutritionist who is knowledgeable about treating HIV infection and is open to using natural therapies. A good place to start is the American Dietetic Association Consumer Nutrition Hotline, 800-366-1655.

Calorie Consumption

Your calorie intake should be 20 to 30 percent higher than the level you needed to maintain weight before you became HIV-positive. If you previously ate a 2,200-a-day diet, 2,900 calories a day may be needed now. But don't make those empty calories, full of fat and artificial ingredients. The six-doughnut breakfast is not a smart shortcut to a higher-calorie diet. Instead, select foods that are healthful and calorie-intensive: brown rice and other grains, lean meat and fish, fruits, avocados, nuts, and seeds (if they aren't hard to digest).

Figure Out Your Calorie Needs

About 30 percent or less of calories should come from fat—some practitioners recommend 25 percent or less because of fat-digestion problems associated with HIV infection that lead to diarrhea. Fifteen percent or more of calories should come from protein. Fifty-five percent should come from carbohydrates, mostly complex carbohydrates such as those found in grains, root vegetables, beans, and legumes.

The FDA's recommended daily calorie intake for men who engage in moderate activity every day (cycling, skiing, tennis, walking 3.5 to 4 miles an hour, weeding, hoeing) is about 3,000. If you are unable to sustain regular moderate activity the suggested calorie intake drops by about 250 to 300 calories a day.

Those with HIV infection are advised to increase basic calorie consumption by about 20 percent over the FDA-recommended levels to maintain weight and by 30 percent to gain weight.

MEN—HIV NEGATIVE	
Age	Calories Needed
15 to 18	3,000
19 to 24	3,000
25 to 50	3,200
51+	2,300

Recommended levels of daily calorie intake for women who engage in regular moderate activity run about 400 to 900 calories a day less than for men, depending on age and body type.

If activity level is low instead of moderate, the calories per day are reduced by about 100. Women who are HIV-positive need to increase calorie intake by 20 percent a day to maintain weight and up to 30 percent for weight gain. Lactating women need to add an extra 500 calories a day; pregnant women, 300.

WOMEN—HIV NEGATIVE	
Age	Calories Needed
19 to 25	2,100
25 to 50	2,300
51+	1,900

Protein Consumption

Taking in sufficient, even extra, protein is essential to stave off wasting and regain lean-muscle mass. The recommended level of protein consumption for an average noninfected woman is 44 to 50 grams a day; men need 45 to 63 grams. Those who are HIV-positive should increase that: Lark Lands, Ph.D., recommends that you multiply your body weight by .7 to find the number of grams of protein you need daily to maintain that weight. When there is increased bodily stress or opportunistic infections, she suggests that the need may increase substantially.

Mary Romeyn, M.D., suggests you increase your consumption over your pre-HIV infection levels by 20 to 30 percent to maintain weight. To regain weight, a rough guideline would be to almost double your daily intake of protein. For more detail, there are handy worksheets in her book, *Nutrition and HIV*, that will guide you through each step.

When eating meats, fish, and dairy foods, which are great protein sources, stick with low-fat varieties. And do not eat flesh that is raw or rare, or unpasteurized dairy products such as imported brie. Ground meat is probably not a good idea, since the meat on the inside of a patty may not be well cooked. Also, avoid raw eggs in sauces, salad dressings, and egg nogs.

Remember also that increased protein levels demand that you drink at least eight glasses of pure water a day in order to help the body process and excrete by-products from metabolized proteins. So although you don't want to drink too much liquid while eating, remember to have a glass of water every hour or two between meals. Overtaxing the kidneys by eating increased amounts of protein and drinking too little water can prove harmful, particularly if you are also taking kidney-stressing medications such as Crixivan.

FAST, FRESH, FLAVORFUL FOOD: R$_X$ RECIPES FOR DIETARY THERAPY

Eating fresh, appealing foods is essential if you are going to retain your appetite—a challenge to many who are HIV-positive. That's why this chapter includes recipes that have been especially designed to provide food that's in tune with the Chinese medicine principles of dietary therapy and tastes delicious.

In addition, many people with HIV infection comment that it becomes physically difficult to cook: These recipes all require minimal preparation time. Other advantages of making your own food:

- Home cooking is cost-effective.
- You can wash vegetables to reduce risk of bacterial infection and cut the risk of debilitating gastrointestinal problems.
- You can enjoy the ritual of nurturing yourself that is so important for the health of the spirit as well as the body.
- You can make sure you get the flavors that appeal to you.

Congee and Soup Recipes

Chinese medicine practitioners often prescribe certain foods to help strengthen and balance Essential Substances. Some contain herbs, others simply use the energetics of the foods themselves. One of the most common foods used for healing is rice, and it is often prescribed in the form of a congee, a boiled-rice porridge that helps prevent disharmonies and strengthens the constitution in those with chronic disorders. You may make a large pot and keep it for several days' meals.

Basic Congee
Basic congee is made with 1 cup white rice (you can use brown rice if you don't have loose stools) and 7 to 9 cups of filtered water, cooked, covered, on low flame for 6 to 8 hours (or use a crock pot). When using vegetables in the

---

**FOOD SAFETY IS A MAJOR ISSUE
FOR PEOPLE WITH HIV INFECTION**

For further information write for the following Food and Drug Administration publications:
- *Food Safety Advice for Persons with AIDS* (publication no. FDA92-2232)
- *Get Hooked on Seafood Safety: Important Information for People with Immune Disorders* (publication no. FDA 93-2267)

Food and Drug Administration
5600 Fishers Lane, HFE-88
Rockville, MD 20857

---

congee, cook them with the rice: Chinese medicine theory is that the vegetables' Qi is distributed through the dish more completely.

General Congees

Add the following ingredients to the basic congee recipe:

- Apricot kernel congee—For asthma, cough, to expel sputum.
- Mung bean congee—Cooling for fevers, general detoxification, for diarrhea and dysentery. Before adding to rice, soak mung beans and then rub off the hard-to-digest shells.
- Aduki bean congee—Removes dampness, benefits edema, gout, and urine retention.
- Carrot congee—For indigestion.
- Leek or garlic congee—Warming and tonifying, good for chronic diarrhea.
- Kidney congee—Generally tonifying, especially for the Kidney. For deficiency symptoms, impotence, weak knees.
- Liver congee—For general Yin Deficiency, anemia, a weak Liver.
- Chicken congee—Good general tonic. Women, add dang gui and ginger.
- Lamb congee—For coldness and poor circulation. Women, add dang gui and ginger.
- Yogurt-honey congee—Benefits Heart and Lung Systems.
- Shan yao (dioscorea) congee—Builds Xue (blood).
- Bai he (bulbous lily) congee—Moistens Lung and strengthens respiration.
- Dried chestnut congee—Kidney tonic, and strengthens the legs.
- Wheat congee—Use wheat in place of half or all the rice to cool the body.
- Sheng jiang (fresh ginger) congee—For general warming, especially on the surface, and neuropathy.

Antiwasting Congees

Add the following ingredients to the basic rice recipe:

- Pickled daikon congee—Benefits digestion and Xue (blood).
- Hi-tech congee with Ultra-clear Sustain from Metagenics—Regulates Spleen Qi, soothes intestines, good for diarrhea, ulcers, indigestion, and irritable bowel (from Abigail Suransky, L.Ac., of Quan Yin).
- Gan jiang (dried ginger) congee—A Spleen Deficiency tonic to help digestion, anorexia, vomiting, and indigestion.
- Mustard green congee—Clears Stomach congestion.
- Beef congee—For weak Spleen, malnutrition, hypoglycemia. Add red ginger to help improve digestion and absorption and make it warming for people who are cold.
- Herbal tonic congee—Add 3 grams of ren shen (ginseng), 6 grams of dang gui (angelica), 6 grams of dang shen (codonopsis), two pieces of hong zao (red dates), 2 pieces of sheng jiang (fresh ginger), and/or 2 pieces of huang qi (astragalus) to tonify the Qi and the Xue and improve digestion.

  For loose stools add to the above 6 grams of lian zi (lotus seeds) and 9 grams of fu ling (poria).

  Herbal congee for diarrhea—6 grams of lian zi (lotus seeds), 3 grams of qian shi (euryale), 3 grams of gan jiang (dried ginger), 6 grams of shan yao (dioscorea), 9 grams of fu ling (poria), 3 grams of dang shen (codonopsis), 2 pieces of hong zao (red dates), plus fresh dates and cinnamon to taste.
- Sweet rice congee—Strengthens the Stomach, tonifies Qi, aids digestion, and is a tonic for diarrhea and vomiting.

Qi Power Chicken Soup

Take this soup to tonify Qi and Xue and strengthen the immune system.

Remove skin from a 3-pound whole chicken. Place whole chicken in a 10-quart pot and cover with water. Bring to boil, then turn down to a simmer.

Add the following:

3 pieces of astragalus (huang qi)
3 grams of codonopsis (dang shen)
3 grams of angelica sinensis (dang gui)
Fresh ginger (sheng jiang), optional
3 grams of ginseng (ren shen), optional

Simmer the chicken, scallions, and ginger for 1½ hours, covered.

When finished, remove the chicken and debone. Return chicken chunks to pot. Add salt to taste if you wish. You can eat all of the herbs except the astragalus, which is too hard to chew.

USING FOODS TO SUPPORT THE SPLEEN

Depending on your current diagnosis, you may want to adjust your dietary intake to reflect these Chinese medicine principles of healing.

For Spleen Qi Deficiency

Avoid:

- Cooling foods such as salads, citrus fruit and juice, and cold, raw tofu
- Too much salt
- Undercooked grains
- Buckwheat and all millet if you are diagnosed as Yang-deficient
- Milk, cheese
- Seaweed, agar
- Too much liquid with meals
- Too much sweet, especially refined sugars

Include:

- Cooked squash, carrot, sweet potato, yam, rutabaga, turnip, leek, onion, pumpkin
- Well-cooked soft rice, sweet rice, and brown rice (unless the deficiency is severe), oats
- Small amounts of chicken, turkey, mutton, beef, and anchovy; venison to fortify the flesh and organs
- Cooked peaches, cherries, and strawberries, dried litchi, figs
- Cardamom, ginger, cinnamon, nutmeg, black pepper
- Kudzu root, arrowroot
- Small amounts of honey and molasses, rice-bran syrup, maple syrup, sugar, or succanat
- Butter, tapioca, and other custards

For Spleen Yang Deficiency

Include the same as for Spleen Qi Deficiency, plus:

- Cayenne
- Dried instead of fresh ginger
- White rice instead of brown rice

Chew all foods well and eat moderate amounts.

For Dampness Associated with Spleen Qi Deficiency

Avoid:

- Excess meat, salt, or sugar
- Dairy products and eggs
- Sardines and octopus
- Tofu, soybeans, olives, and pine nuts
- Cucumbers and spinach

Include: the same as all the above, plus:

- Aduki beans
- Alfalfa
- Barley
- Chicken
- Corn
- Garlic
- Mushrooms
- Mustard greens
- Rye
- Shrimp
- Scallions

For Spleen Qi Deficiency with Damp Cold

Avoid:

- Red meat
- Raw vegetables
- Fruit juices
- Dairy

Include:

- Three quarters of your calories from grains and legumes
- About 12 ounces of lean, white meat a week
- Cooked vegetables of all types

NUTRITIONAL SUPPLEMENTS

Although you should be able to get all the nutrition you need from a well-balanced diet, even the most conscientious among us are hard pressed to protect ourselves against the daily wear and tear of pollution, pesticide and chemically contaminated foods, and overrefined food products. When you combine these factors with the effects of HIV and related infections, I believe it is important to take a carefully designed regime of vitamins and minerals under the supervision of a nutritionist, Chinese medicine practitioner, or Western doctor. High doses of some vitamins and minerals can interfere with drug action, become toxic, or have a harmful effect on the absorption and use of other vitamins and minerals, so you don't want to start dosing yourself without careful examination of the problems that might arise.

You may find that both Chinese and Western practitioners suggest differing levels of or types of supplementation. The wisest course for any person interested in taking charge of her health is to carefully research and read all opinions and make a choice to follow a course that is well balanced. In this section, in addition to my own recommendations, I present the recommendations of two HIV practitioners whom I respect but who do not always agree with one another: Lark Lands, Ph.D., and Mary Romeyn, M.D. I urge you to explore their perspectives further (see Appendix 5).

And now, here are the guidelines for nutritional supplementation that I recommend to my clients.

- **Acidophilus**—One fourth to $1/2$ teaspoon three times per day between meals. Use a refrigerated powdered acidophilus product such as Natren brand Pro-Bionate or Maxidophilus, Megadophilus, or Primadophilus.
- **A multivitamin, multimineral supplement**—In powder (usually in capsule), not pill form; it is much easier to digest and absorb. Make sure it supplies selenium and chromium.
- **Essential fatty acids**—One tablespoon a day of organic flax, raw sesame, or evening primrose oil to help promote production of prostaglandins. They should be refrigerated before and after opening to prevent rancidity.
- **Caretenoids or beta-carotene**—25,000+ units per day, depending on your condition and with approval and supervision of your practitioner.[5] Do not take Vitamin A—it appears to be unwise for those who are HIV-

positive. For a more direct, and perhaps healthier, supplementation, every other day drink a 4-ounce glass of fresh organic carrot juice made at home, from carrots washed in a dilute solution of Clorox. More is not better in this case: There appear to be other factors in carrots themselves that, when taken in large quantities over time, produce negative side effects.

- **Vitamin E**—800 to 1,200 IU of alpha tocopherol a day. This antioxidant has been found to benefit the body in numerous ways, from easing PMS symptoms to stalling Alzheimer's-related memory loss. Deficiency can lead to peripheral neuropathy. Furthermore, there is some indication that E increases AZT's effectiveness, and supplementation of 800 IUs a day was also shown to increase cell-mediated immunity in HIV-negative elderly.

- **Vitamin C**—Six grams a day or more of the ascorbate form of the nutrient; I like a fizzy powder, such as Wholesale Nutrition's C-Salts. If you experience gas or loose stools, reduce the dose immediately until you find a comfortable level. Some people can't take vitamin C because it is too acidic and causes mouth sores. In addition, people with Spleen Qi Deficiency and diarrhea should take Vitamin C only if their Chinese medicine practitioner prescribes it. C works as an antioxidant, and when the body is under stress or fighting infection the need for C increases. Vitamin C research suggests that a deficiency can decrease the immune system's ability to fight off bacterial infection.

- **Garlic capsules or pills**—Use as directed for candidiasis.

The B Vitamins

I don't usually make specific recommendations for taking the B vitamins, since they are included in your multivitamins, but there is a lot of interesting information about them in relationship to HIV infection. I pass this along so that you and your practitioner can determine when and if additional supplements are necessary.

Levels of the various B vitamins appear to be lowered in people who are HIV-positive, and supplementation may be an important component of battling weight loss and reduced strength.

- B-12 deficiencies, found in almost a quarter of HIV-positive people, particularly those with absorption problems, may contribute to neurological dysfunction and anemia. In addition, Johns Hopkins University and the Janeway Child Health Care Centre in Canada reported findings from the analysis of data on 312 gay men who had their blood sampled in 1984 and were tracked twice yearly until the end of 1993, when the micronutrient analysis was done. Those who had the largest deficiencies in B-12 and E also had the greatest amount of disease progression.[6] Optimal levels of supplementation aren't really known. Some B-vitamin supplements have up to 500 micrograms of B-12—what you don't need is passed in the urine.

• Vitamin B-6 deficiencies were found in 35 percent of HIV-positive people in one study, and the authors speculated that lack of sufficient fresh fruits and vegetables in the diet is the main cause. Deficiency may also arise as a result of endocrine responses to the presence of HIV (specifically, an increase in tumor necrosis factor) and a reduction in lean-muscle mass, where B-6 is usually stored. Medication for tuberculosis—particularly Isoniazid—also produces a B-6 deficiency. The results of B-6 deficiency include altered neuropsychiatric function: A 1994 study found that HIV-positive men who increased or maintained sufficient B-6 levels reported significantly less psychological distress than those who were B-6–deficient.[7] However, several studies indicate over-supplementation with B-6 may produce peripheral neuropathy, a numbness or tingling in the fingers and toes, and HIV-positive people should be particularly cautious.[8] Supplements of 20 to 50 milligrams a day are often recommended if you're taking Isoniazid; around 20 milligrams a day for HIV-positive people is generally sufficient in the absence of other factors.

• Vitamin B-1 (thiamine) converts carbohydrates into energy and is an important part of an antiwasting diet. Red meats, grains, nuts, and legumes are all good sources. In addition, supplementing with a multivitamin provides an extra few milligrams, and a separate B-vitamin supplement can contain more than 50 milligrams.

• Vitamin B-2 (riboflavin) is involved in the metabolism of amino acids that build proteins. Deficiencies can arise if you are taking antinausea drugs such as Compazine, mood elevators such as Elavil, or amitriptyline, which is sometimes used to treat HIV-related foot pain. Around 3 milligrams, found in most multivitamins, will help prevent deficiency, although B-vitamin supplements pack up to 100 milligrams.

• Folic acid plays an important role in manufacturing red blood cells and in maintaining healthy neurological processes. There is also an indication, according to Lark Lands and others, that 10 milligrams a day helps ward off cervical dysplasia, which is often associated with the development of cancer. The deficiency arises for several reasons: Faulty digestion and absorption short-change the body; there is some evidence that AZT reduces folate levels; Bactrim and Septra, two names for a medication prescribed to prevent or control *Pneumocystis carinii* pneumonia (PCP), are folate blockers. One to 2 milligrams a day may help prevent deficiency, and leafy vegetables, eggs, legumes, yeast, and organ meats are good food sources.

• Other B vitamins—biotin, niacin, pantothenic acid—are rarely deficient, and routine multiple vitamins offer sufficient supplies.

MARY ROMEYN'S BASIC ADVICE

• Take N-acetyl cysteine (NAC). An antioxidant amino acid, NAC provides an important component of the peptide glutathione and is thought to help block HIV replication and increase CD4+ counts independent of increases in the glutathione levels. Dr. Romeyn recommends NAC despite confusing results of certain studies.[9]

• Use flavor-enhancing supplements that emphasize natural flavors and smells. Salt and sweet often remain appealing when subtler flavors are hard to discern, so don't hesitate to make food appealing by relying on these tastes, as long as you are not on a low-sodium diet and are not being treated for blood sugar–related medical problems. In Chinese medicine small amounts of salt and sugar are important parts of a balanced diet.

• Don't take zinc. Dr. Romeyn feels there are four convincing studies that demonstrate it has a negative effect in people with HIV infection.

• Back off vitamin A in light of a study by Barbara Weiser at the Wadsworth Center in Albany, New York, showing that it is not needed for HIV patients in this country. "I've cut back my recommendations to fifteen milligrams of beta-carotene a day," says Dr. Romeyn. "I don't want to risk harming anyone and there's no evidence that it helps."

ADDITIONAL SELF-CARE FOR AN ANTIWASTING PROGRAM

In order to mount an effective antiwasting campaign you will want to use other tools such as exercise, stress reduction and meditation, control of addictions, and Chinese herbs and acupuncture. They all reinforce your dietary efforts and offer you a solid opportunity to maintain your strength.

Exercise

Exercise to build lean-muscle mass is an essential component of any antiwasting or weight-gaining program. Not only does exercise in general help ease depression, thus giving the immune system a boost, but it also strengthens basic immune responses, and weight training builds lean-muscle mass.

This is particularly important for women, according to a Tufts University assistant professor of medicine, Ronenn Roubenoff, M.D.: "Women appear to be losing lean mass faster than men, although we don't yet know why." The answers may emerge eventually; Tufts is in the middle of a five-year project, Nutrition for Life, which is studying the effects of diet, exercise, and weight loss on the health of 500 HIV-positive adults and children. The Tufts study, funded by the National Institutes of Health, is the first long-term investigation of HIV infection and nutrition to examine a broad patient mix, including women, minorities, and intravenous-drug users.

LARK LANDS'S BASIC SUPPLEMENT RECOMMENDATIONS

- Multivitamin-multimineral—Made from advanced forms of the minerals (citrates, picolinates, ascorbates, etc.) and B vitamins.
- Multiple antioxidant—Containing beta-carotene, selenium, vitamin E, glutathione, etc.
- Acidophilus—2 to 4 capsules with each meal.
- Alpha-lipoic acid—300 to 600 milligrams (mg) a day of this antioxidant.
- Ascorbic acid/ascorbate—2 to 6 grams a day.
- Beta-carotene—50,000 to 200,000 units a day.
- B-12—1,000 micrograms through nasal gel or injection two to seven times a week.
- Coenzyme Q_{10}—30 to 300 mg a day.
- Vitamin E—800 to 1,000 IU a day.
- Essential fatty acids—Taken as evening primrose oil or borage or grapeseed oil, 240 to 1,440 mg a day.
- Glutamine—10 to 15 grams a day.
- N-acetyl cysteine (NAC)—1,800 to 5,400 mg a day.
- Selenium—400 to 800 mg a day. If you are getting selenium in your multiple vitamin you may have enough. Over 1,000 mg a day may be toxic.
- Zinc—25 to 50 mg a day. A multiple vitamin may supply enough; more than 100 mg a day over the long term may be toxic.

Other studies have already been completed that demonstrated the use of weight lifting in building immune strength: A study at the Naval Medical Center in San Diego, California, found that HIV-positive men who did regular weight lifting had less of a decline in their mean CD4+ counts than did nonexercisers (a 2.1 percent decline over two years as compared to a 2.7 percent decline over the same length of time). Runners who could cover a mile in less than eight minutes and ran three times a week fared far, far worse than either weight lifters or nonexercisers: They saw a 6.4 percent drop in their CD4+ counts over two years. All study participants were taking anti-HIV therapy.

While it appears that strenuous aerobic exercise might be depleting to the body—which conforms precisely to Chinese medicine's concepts of exercise—Qi Gong exercises help strengthen your constitution and increase flexibility while boosting your muscle strength. For complete information on Qi Gong and a complete exercise program, see Chapter 9.

Meditation and Stress Release

Stress is a part of the fabric of everyday life; add to it the stress of living with HIV infection, being sick, and worrying about your finances and your health care, and you've got a formula for stress-related illnesses and depression. Using Qi Gong meditation and yoga along with a wide spectrum of Western stress-relief techniques is essential if you are to optimize your health and stay in control of your well-being. For meditation routines and resources for finding out about other alternatives, see Chapter 9.

Substance-Abuse Treatment

Nutritional support and weight-gaining efforts will not help you stay as healthy as you would like or manage HIV infection as well as you might if you are still struggling with drug or alcohol dependency. The immune and organ systems are severely compromised by the use of recreational drugs or overuse of prescription mind-alerting medication. Women especially are overmedicated with tranquilizers and antidepressants. For a program to help you balance addictive patterns see page 180.

7

⊙

The Basic HIV+
Herbal Therapy Program:
Prescription for Enhanced
Balance and Strength

I was diagnosed almost nine years ago and have had only a couple of
bouts of illness. In all that time I have never used any Western
antiviral medicine. Instead I use herbs to support my immune system
and help keep my marrow strong. I think this has been the key to my
long-term healthiness—that and the attention I pay to my diet and
overall frame of mind. Some day they'll figure out exactly what these
herbs do—but until then, all I need to know is that they work for me.
—Karen G., AIDS counselor and former schoolteacher,
diagnosed in 1991

Have you ever walked into a Chinese herbalists' shop with its hundreds of drawers and glass jars filled with potent plants, animal extracts, and
minerals? It certainly looks mysterious, but in reality it is a well-ordered laboratory where the healing wisdom of the past 2,000 years waits to be distilled
into a prescription tailored to remedy your individual disharmonies. In fact,
the herbs and herb formulas that your practitioner or herbalist prescribes are
potent medicine and should not be taken on a whim or without supervision.
Few herbs from the vast pharmacopoeia of Chinese medicine are recommended to be used as over-the-counter remedies. That's why it's so important
to put yourself in the hands of a well-trained and experienced professional
who is capable of diagnosing you accurately and treating you effectively. And
I strongly recommend that you see your Chinese medicine practitioner regularly while you are taking the herbs so she can monitor your responses to the
treatment.

In exploring the use of herbal therapy, keep in mind that there are three
important distinctions between Western drugs and Chinese herbal medicine.
First, in Chinese herbal therapy the concept of how herbs interact so that they
effectively counter illness and restore harmony is based on the philosophy of

the Tao—that a well-balanced whole is formed by the unity of opposites. Second, Chinese herbal medicine uses only naturally occurring ingredients. For example, there is no such thing as prescribing a synthetic hormone such as progestin to replace the body's own progesterone. Last but perhaps most important, when prescribed by a knowledgeable practitioner, herbs rarely have negative side effects of any consequence. So let's take a look inside those mysterious-looking jars of strangely named herbs and find out exactly how they work to restore harmony to the Organ Systems and Essential Substances.

HOW HERBS ARE DESCRIBED

Herbs are characterized by temperature, taste, and direction. The impact of each aspect must be weighed when determining the proper herbal remedy for a specific disharmony.

Temperature. An herb may be hot, cold, warm, cool, or neutral. If a disease is considered hot, then a cool or cold herb is needed. If the disharmony is cold, then a warming herb is required.

Taste. An herb may be characterized as acrid, sweet, bitter, sour, or salty. Substances with none of these qualities are labeled bland (they sure are!). Each of these qualities has its own unique therapeutic impact on Essential Substances. Acrid herbs disperse and move; sweet ones tonify and harmonize. Bitter herbs drain and dry. Sour herbs are astringent and prevent or reverse the normal leakage of fluids and energy. Salty herbs purge. And bland herbs take out dampness and promote urination.

Direction. The therapeutic impact of an herb can also be measured in terms of the direction that it moves Essential Substances. Some herbs cause the Qi to rise and float (move upward and outward), some cause it to fall and sink (move downward and inward).

HERBAL THERAPY IN THE HIV+ PROGRAM

The herbal formulas I use in our program were developed by blending the wisdom of ancient Chinese herbalists with modern scientific insights into the pharmacological effects of herbs. We began systematically studying the impact of various herbs on HIV in 1986–87, when the Brion Herb Corporation, a Chinese herbal company, donated approximately $30,000 worth of herbal formulas in the form of granulated herbal powders to the San Francisco AIDS Alternative Healing Project (which I cofounded) and Qingcai Zhang, M.D., of the Oriental Healing Arts Institute (OHAI) in Long Beach, California. Together we developed the protocol (a detailed treatment plan) for a study of the effects of herbs on people with HIV/AIDS.

In that first six-month study we followed 23 people who had been diagnosed as HIV-positive (most of those who had progressed to AIDS were taking

---

POSSIBLE NEGATIVE EFFECTS OF CHINESE HERBS

One question that comes up all the time is "Do Chinese herbs have any negative interactions with Western drugs used to treat HIV infection?" To date we have seen none.

Generally, prescribed herbs and herbal formulas are safe and without unpleasant or negative effects. However, negative reactions are, of course, possible to any organic substance or combination of substances. And HIV infection often makes a person more sensitive to herbs than other people are, just as it makes them more sensitive to drug therapy.

Digestive upset is the most common negative reaction and it usually lasts for only a couple of days, until the body adjusts to the high fiber content of the new treatment. However, if the digestive upset persists more than a few days or is severe, measures should be taken promptly to ease the reaction.

More significant problems arise with specific herbs that are not safe if you happen to have a particular disease or disorder. For example, those with liver disease should avoid some herbs. While they may not cause problems for people with a healthy liver, if there is already liver damage, they can further injure the tissue. If you have liver disease, always ask your practitioner or herbalist about possible contraindications.

The best way to avoid side effects or to alleviate them is by using practitioners who are well trained and who know you and your medical history.

AZT) and six who had chronic fatigue immune dysfunction syndrome. During the study we measured the effects of 28 herbal formulas, monitoring their effect by using Chinese medicine diagnosis and blood tests to check platelet and white and red blood cell counts; liver, kidney, and heart function; and the presence of the p24 antigen. The University of California–San Francisco processed the blood samples in their laboratories.

At first we were simply feeling our way through this process—carefully looking for clinical indications of what was working and adjusting our treatments depending on the results we observed. Pretty soon, though, we had honed in on six formulas that seemed most effective. And we began using other substances that the clients found helpful. For example, one young man who'd been diagnosed a year earlier was suffering from severe anemia and required two to three blood transfusions a week. He was very cold and unresponsive. Dr. Zhang prescribed sliced deer antler for him and he became more energetic and needed fewer transfusions. So we decided to give deer antler to others in the study who were also anemic and cold. That's how we learned that marrow-strengthening agents are an important part of herbal therapy for HIV infection.

In another instance, a visiting scientist, Dr. Chen of Shanghai, supplied us with an enema made from a traditional herbal formula for diarrhea, which we used with some success with those suffering from cryptosporidium-related diarrhea.

We added a concentrated form of *Ganoderma lucidum* mushroom, donated by BioHerb, Inc., and found it boosted people's energy levels dramatically. During this program it became more and more evident that Toxic Heat was a trigger for HIV-related symptoms and associated disharmonies. There is a category of Chinese herbs known traditionally as Clear Heat Clean Toxin—no surprise that it would make sense to use these against the epidemic factor Toxic Heat. We started using a formula of antiviral, heat-clearing herbs from this category in all the base formulas.

We were able to use Western scientific discoveries to make the formulas even more effective. Western research had shown that only a few Clear Heat Clean Toxin herbs have any anti-HIV effect in vitro, and even fewer have a strong virus-killing effect.[1] Therefore, in developing immune-strengthening HIV herbal formulas, we used only those herbs that had the strongest virucidal effects, not only for HIV but also for herpes, hepatitis viruses, and other viruses.[2] We also included components such as the fungus *Cordyceps sineusis,* which is antibacterial and is used in China for its anticancer properties.

As we proceeded, always refining our formulas, we were faced with the problem of how to measure and evaluate the participants' responses. This was the beginning of the ongoing debate about how to assess the most common response of people taking Chinese medicine treatments for HIV infection: "I have more energy." We decided the clearest empirical measure available was to evaluate the degree of change in the study subjects' daily activities: Ten of the original 29 participants were unable to work at the outset of the study. Six months later, at the close of the study, all but one participant was employed or doing consistent volunteer work.

At the end of that first casual, observational study by the San Francisco AIDS Alternative Healing Project, the Quan Yin Healing Arts Center, and the Oriental Healing Arts Institute in 1988, I approached Dr. Subhuti Dharmananda of the Institute for Traditional Medicine (ITM) in Portland, Oregon, and we agreed to conduct the Quan Yin Herbal Program for People with AIDS. ITM, which manufactures herb formulas, agreed to supply the test formulas to Quan Yin at reduced cost in exchange for Quan Yin's collaboration. In one month, Quan Yin Healing Arts Center recruited 90 clients from the Quan Yin Acupuncture and Herb Center. As part of the protocol we developed monitoring questionnaires, as well as a way to draw blood that would yield consistent lab results. When the two-year cooperation ended in 1990, the Quan Yin Herbal Program had formally enrolled and followed more than 600 people. Over time we went through several different herbal formulations designed by ITM and a company producing herbal formulas called Health Concerns, ultimately using one called Composition A tailored to treat HIV-positive people. In addition, Quan Yin had treated many more HIV-positive people with a combination of acupuncture and herbs. I presented the results in Beijing at the First International Conference on Viral Hepatitis and AIDS in 1991.

In early 1991, I began work on another new formula based on insights gathered through observational and clinical experience with more than 2,000 clients at Quan Yin since the beginning of the HIV/AIDS epidemic. Health Concerns agreed to support its development. After a 16-week trial period, Health Concerns began distributing two formulas I developed, Enhance and Clear Heat. The next spring, in conjunction with Health Concerns founder Andrew Gaeddert, I designed Marrow Plus, based on my work with people with cancer and HIV infection. This formula—designed specifically for people who were receiving chemotherapy or AZT and had low blood cell counts—can also benefit those who have HIV- and drug-related anemia.

In 1992–93 I was the coinvestigator on a double-blind placebo-controlled study at San Francisco General Hospital. Using IGM-1—a formula designed from Enhance and Clear Heat—we observed that gastrointestinal and neurological symptoms improved and fatigue lessened. We also saw a trend toward improved sleep patterns and lessening of pain.

Since that early study there have been many more refinements in the herbal formulas and I have designed Source Qi for treatment of chronic diarrhea. This process of inquiry and study led to the herbal protocol outlined below that is used in my clinic and by many practitioners in the United States and around the world today.

HIV+ HERBAL PROTOCOL

The formulas I developed for regulating immunity and suppressing Toxic Heat, Enhance and Tremella American Ginseng, and specifically for suppressing Toxic Heat, Clear Heat, are based on Chinese medicine herbal therapies known as Fu Zheng and Jiedu/Qiuxie. *Fu Zheng* means "restoring normality," and it is used in China to tonify Qi and Xue and to increase disease resistance, normalize various bodily functions, and regulate the immune system of people with cancer. We've adopted it to treat chronic immune dysfunction associated with chronic viral disease and to decrease or eliminate the side effects of Western anti-HIV medications and of chemotherapy and radiation.

Jiedu/Qiuxie therapy is used to clear toxins and heat from the body. These herbs are very powerful and are used only in combination with Fu Zheng therapy, which ameliorates the potential side effects of antitoxins. Traditionally, these herbs have been used in China to destroy cancers and to treat Heat Toxin diseases, which we now know include viral and bacterial infections.

Basic Herbal Pill Formulas

The basic herbal pill formulas used at Chicken Soup Chinese Medicine Clinic and Quan Yin to treat most people with HIV infection are Enhance, Tremella American Ginseng, and Source Qi.

> I want to stress that although many practitioners use the herbal formula pills that I have designed, as well as the many other pill herbs outlined below, your practitioner does not have to use these to provide effective treatment. As long as the basic therapeutic principals are followed—support the Spleen and Stomach, counter Toxic Heat, strengthen the Marrow, tonify the Kidney, regulate Liver Qi, tonify Xue, Yin and Yang, and support digestion—your practitioner's individualized herbal formulas and treatments can be equally efficacious.

- For tonification and immunoregulation and antiviral action, the base formulas are Enhance and Tremella American Ginseng.
- For predominant Stomach/Spleen Deficiency, Toxic Heat, Dampness, Xue Deficiency, and need to tonify the Center: Enhance.
- For predominant Yin Deficiency symptoms such as dry skin, red skin, reddish tongue color, and heat sensations such as flushing: Tremella American Ginseng.
- For predominant Spleen Yang Deficiency with diarrhea or loose stools: Source Qi.

Formulas Used in Conjunction with Basic Herbal Protocol

In addition to the basic herbal protocol, several other formulas are often used to individualize treatment for people with HIV infection.

- For clearing heat and removing toxins, and to treat increased viral load and viral or bacterial infections: Clear Heat.
- To tonify and vitalize the Xue (blood), for drug-related anemia, drug toxicity, and decreased platelet and white and red blood cell counts: Marrow Plus.
- To tonify Spleen Yang and remove cold and damp and to strengthen digestion; for possible treatment of severe diarrhea with undigested food, parasites, and cryptosporidium: Source Qi.
- For regulation and tonification of Qi and Xue (blood) and to treat PMS, hormonal imbalances, menstrual cramps, and hepatitis: Woman's Balance.
- To regulate Qi and vitalize the Xue (blood), used for chronic hepatitis and impaired liver function: Ecliptex.

For additional herb formulas in pill form that are commonly used in treating specific disharmonies, see Appendixes 2 and 3.

Advantages of the HIV+ Herbal Pill Protocol

- The pills cost less than individually mixed formulas. When herbal formulas are made in large quantities, the cost per dose decreases.
- Following the treatment regime with pills is easier than cooking up individual batches of herbs, which is time-consuming, and for some people off-putting.
- The herbs are formulated specifically to treat persons with HIV infection and chronic immune dysfunction associated with chronic viral disease.
- The dosages are more potent than those in raw herb mixtures, because properly prepared pills deliver the full power of herbs. However, you must make sure that the herb company you use is preparing the herbs in a traditional way—such as frying them in honey or cooking them in rice wine—before converting them into pill form.
- Increased efficacy. All the herb formulas that I design are tested at Quan Yin and in other practices before they go into general distribution.
- The use of basic formulas is safe for those without a nearby practitioner. While the best treatment is to have a Chinese traditional medicine practitioner who has been trained in managing HIV infection, the second-best option is to have the basic herbal formulas available to physicians worldwide who can then consult with experts by phone, fax, or mail if necessary. We urge you to limit your use of herbs to the basic formulas we recommend if you are not under the care of a knowledgeable Chinese medicine practitioner.

Advantages of Individualized Herbal Formulas

Practitioners tend to use formulas made from individual herbs or their extracts or powders for acute problems that have changeable symptoms. Although herbal pills may be convenient, when a client has a viral cold, flu, herpes outbreak, or acute sinus infection, it is often more efficacious to use strong herbal teas, or soups (as they are called in Chinese). They can be designed to treat an individual's exact symptoms.

In very complicated cases for which I do not have an herbal pill, I will combine raw herbs into formulas in conjunction with herbal pills. That's why a number of my clients with AIDS, cancer, and CFIDS cook up raw herbal formulas at home to take in conjunction with basic pill formulas such as Enhance or Tremella American Ginseng. Some people also believe that the process of preparing the herbs from scratch is part of the healing process and they are more comfortable with the raw formulas.

HERBS USED IN HIV/AIDS PROGRAMS

Herbs That Affect Immune Functions

The following herbs are *Qi tonics,* which increase energy and reduce the effects of chronic infection. They are used in Chinese medicine to strengthen the body's overall energy.

Astragalus *(huang qi)*

Astragalus membranaceus is used as a tonic herb, particularly for the Spleen and Lung, and is an important ingredient in herbal formulas used to strengthen Qi. It is a Fu Zheng herb and is found in Enhance, Tremella American Ginseng, Marrow Plus, and Source Qi. For HIV-positive–related disharmonies, it is particularly important because it

- Increases appetite and aids in digestion and absorption of food.
- Stops both night sweats and day sweats.
- Helps with healing of injured tissue.

CURRENT RESEARCH. According to Western research, astragalus has immune restorative capabilities in both the cell-mediated and humoral aspects of the immune system. Several Chinese studies have found that it increases the red blood cell count. It has been studied for its anticancer effects.[3] In a Chinese study using astragalus, survival rates were increased from 28 percent to 71 percent in people with liver or lung cancer.[4] In another Chinese study of chronic active hepatitis, 18 of 31 participants had their liver function return to normal.[5] Astragalus has the ability to stimulate interferon to reduce the viral symptoms of the common cold.[6] In combination with other herbs, it helps fight infection and builds up resistance to viruses and bacteria.[7] Astragalus also aids in the discharge of pus from hard-to-heal wounds. In animal studies, it has also had the effect of lowering blood pressure.[8]

APPLICATIONS. The principal applications of astragalus are prevention of cold and flu; treatment of chronic kidney inflammation (nephritis) to decrease edema and protein in the urine;[9] immune regulation.

Atractylodes *(bai zhu)*

Atractylodes macrocephala, or white atractylodes, is another important Qi tonic herb. It is used to tonify—strengthen—the Spleen and the Stomach Systems and improve digestion; it is also used to remove dampness. Atractylodes is a Qi tonic and a Fu Zheng herb and appears in formulas such as Bu Zhong Yi Qi Tang (Central Chi Tea), Si Jun Zi Tang (Four Gentlemen Tea), Source Qi, and Enhance. The chemical constituents include atractylone, actractylol, and vitamin A.

CURRENT RESEARCH. Researchers in China have reported that atractylodes can increase white blood cell counts, and it is used in formulas that are designed to strengthen immune function.[10] Furthermore, this herb has been demonstrated to lower elevated blood sugar and prevent excess glycogen concentration in the liver.[11] It is also used to reduce platelet aggregation that can lead to the formation of blood clots.[12]

People with HIV infection sometimes suffer from a blood-clotting disorder called idiopathic thrombocytopenia, a reduction in blood platelets of unknown cause. They should consult a doctor before taking this herb. However, because of the way Chinese herbs are combined, this potential hazard is likely to be reduced. In fact, at Quan Yin, we've seen that people with HIV infection who take herbal formulas containing this herb actually experience a stabilization of their platelets.

APPLICATIONS. Atractylodes is used in formulas to help increase body weight and muscle strength. It is also found in formulas for reducing swelling, easing diarrhea, treating Qi Deficiency, resolving heart disharmonies, and enhancing the immune system. It also tonifies the Spleen and Stomach.

Ganoderma *(ling zhi)*

Ganoderma lucidum is a fungus (mushroom), also known as the reishi mushroom, whose active ingredients are primarily found in the spores. The various types contain active chemicals such as ergosterol, coumanin, and mannitol. Traditionally, the red ling zhi variety is considered the most powerful.[13] This Fu Zheng herb is a main ingredient in many important HIV herb formulas, including Enhance, Composition A, and Resist. In addition to being a Qi tonic, it calms the spirit and tonifies Xue.

CURRENT RESEARCH. Ganoderma contains highly active polysaccharides, which appear to have a potent immune-regulating effect.[14]

APPLICATIONS. Ganoderma protects the liver from damage,[15] reduces the symptoms of hepatitis,[16] and lowers liver enzyme levels (elevated levels are associated with impaired liver function).[17] It also helps regulate the immune system (the Japanese and Chinese have focused on its anticancer properties).[18] And it helps with breathing, especially for those with asthma, and eases insomnia.[19]

Licorice Root *(gan cao)*

Glycyrrhiza glabra, or licorice root, is included in many formulas to harmonize the blend of herbs so that their effects can enter the channels and be transported to the Organ Systems as needed. Licorice root is a component in formulas used in the Basic HIV+ Herbal Therapy Program: Enhance, and Tremella American Ginseng.

CURRENT RESEARCH. The effect of licorice root on the immune system has been reported in several studies from Japan and China. They indicate it may act as an antiviral agent for people with HIV infection[20] and in anticancer therapy.[21] It also has properties that appear to be antiviral for hepatitis B. A German study showed a success rate of 30 to 40 percent in treatment of chronic viral hepatitis B, against which little has been found to be effective.[22]

APPLICATIONS. Licorice root is traditionally used to strengthen the Spleen and help with weak digestion. It stops pain and spasms, has an antitoxicity effect, and is often used as an anti-inflammatory in the treatment of arthritis and gastric ulcers. It is also used to treat sore throats and immune dysfunction.

Licorice can be toxic; over a long period of time, high doses may trigger high blood pressure, reduce thyroid function, and have other side effects. Chinese herbal formulas contain very little glycyrrhiza, but even so it should be taken only under the supervision of a qualified health-care provider.

Codonopsis *(dang shen)*

Codonopsis pilosula is used because of its tonifying and harmonizing effect on the Stomach and the Spleen. The Chinese have also reported that it helps T cell transformation and increases the red blood cell count.

APPLICATIONS. Codonopsis is particularly important for people with HIV infection because it helps to increase appetite and weight and controls diarrhea. It also helps ease chronic sputum-producing cough, which is associated with the HIV-related Spleen deficiency.

Yin Tonics

Yin tonics are used to provide strength and balance when the body is profoundly depleted and becoming dry and inflexible.

American Ginseng *(xi yang shen)*

The root of *Panax quinquefolium* produces a sedative effect on the brain at the same time that it excites the central nervous system. It is often used to restore energy after a fever and for clearing the lungs. The main ingredients are panaquilon and saponins.

APPLICATIONS. When used in combination with Tremella, American Ginseng fights viral infection and strengthens the immune system.

Ligustrum *(nu zhen zi)*

The fruit of *Ligustrum lucidum* acts as a tonic for people with HIV infection and many forms of cancer who suffer from wasting syndromes. It also tonifies the Kidney and Liver Yin. The main ingredients have been identified as oleanolic acid, oleic acid, linoleic acid, fructoses, glucoses, and mannitol.[23]

CURRENT RESEARCH. Ligustrum strengthens the Kidney Jing and Yin and is important for its antibacterial effects and ability to help increase the white blood cell count.

APPLICATIONS. This herb is used to alleviate vertigo, low-back pain, ringing in the ears, and low fever from tuberculosis.

Tremella *(bai mu er)*

Tremella fuciformis is used to counter emaciation and to ease respiratory problems. The main ingredients have been identified as vitamin B, and traces of minerals including iron, calcium, sulfur, phosphate, magnesium, and potassium.

APPLICATIONS. This herb is used to nourish the Stomach and moisten the Lung Systems and so is often used to treat consumption, dry coughs, and tuberculosis. It is also useful in combination with American ginseng in treating chronic viral infections that have created Heat Deficiency patterns and Yin Deficiency, such as happens in HIV-related disorders.

Astringent Herbs

Astringent herbs help ease dampness and draw out toxins. These are important qualities for those with HIV/AIDS because of the role of Spleen Qi Deficiency and dampness (and damp heat) in many of the associated symptoms such as chronic diarrhea, candidiasis, fever, nausea, abdominal pain, and headaches.

Ginkgo Leaf *(yin guo ye)*

The *Ginkgo biloba* leaf has traditionally been used as an astringent herb to preserve the lungs, calm wheezing, and stop chest pain. Recently it has been used for angina pectoris, to lower elevated cholesterol levels, restore long-term memory loss, and ease depression.

CURRENT RESEARCH. It has been shown that one to three weeks' treatment with *Ginkgo biloba* extract can improve symptoms of memory loss, anxiety, lack of concentration, compromised psychomotor skills, and headache. The studies demonstrating these effects were based on a standardized *Ginkgo biloba* extract, 50:1, not whole Ginkgo leaves.

APPLICATIONS. Used for treatment of mental impairment and dementia associated with HIV infection, and several forms of opportunistic infection, including toxoplasmosis. As a lung remedy it is useful in the treatment of *Pneumocystis carinii* pneumonia. It can also be used to treat cardiovascular disease and problems associated with vascular impairment such as ringing in the ears, vertigo, cramps, intermittent claudication, and penile erectile dysfunction.[24]

Schizandra *(wu wei zi)*

This fruit, *Schizandra chinensis,* acts as an intestinal astringent, and works as both a Qi and a Kidney tonic. For treatment of HIV-associated disharmonies, schizandra is used in Enhance. In Tremella American Ginseng it helps decrease sweating and promotes secretion of body fluids. In Ecliptex it is used for its ability to protect the liver and counter the effects of hepatitis. Schizandra Dreams is a modern formula designed to ease insomnia. Tian Wang Bu Xin Wang is a traditional formula used for similar purposes.

CURRENT RESEARCH. Chinese researchers have found that schizandra decreases elevated liver enzyme levels, which are associated with liver disease, in almost three quarters of people studied in an average of 25 days.[25] It also helps counter fatigue and stress.

APPLICATIONS. Used as an intestinal astringent, schizandra helps control diarrhea; it also has a soothing effect upon the Shen. It also inhibits sweating, generates fluids, stops coughs, and quiets the spirit.

Antiviral, Antibacterial, Antitoxin Herbs

Most of the herbs that have these functions are in the Clear Heat Clean Toxin category and are used in China as antiviral, antibacterial agents. They are important elements in the fight against Toxic Heat and the symptoms associated with HIV-related disharmonies.

Isatis Leaf *(da qing ye)* and Isatis Root *(ban lan gen)*

Isatis tinctoria is antiviral and antibacterial. Its main chemical component is indigo.

CURRENT RESEARCH. Studies demonstrate that isatis is effective in treating viral hepatitis, herpes, and viral meningitis. Isatis root is often included in anti-cancer formulas and in treatment of chronic myelogenous leukemia.[26]

APPLICATIONS. In China isatis leaf and isatis root are used frequently to treat serious bacterial infections such as shigella, salmonella, streptococcus, and staphylococcus. They play an essential role in the basic HIV+ Herbal Therapy

Program's formulas Enhance and Tremella American Ginseng and in Clear Heat, which is often used as an adjunct to the basic formulas.

Viola *(zi hua di ding)*

Viola yedoensis is potent Clear Heat Clean Toxin. In the base formulas for the HIV+ Herbal Therapy program—Enhance and Tremella, American Ginseng—and in Clear Heat viola works as an antiviral, antibacterial agent. Its main chemical constituents are cerotic acid and saponin.

CURRENT RESEARCH. Studies at the University of California–Davis and Hong Kong University found that viola was the strongest anti-HIV agent—at least in a test tube—among many herbs they studied. The World Health Organization also recommended viola as a cost-effective antiviral against HIV.[27] Viola also has antibacterial properties, particularly against HIV-related opportunistic infections associated with streptococcus, pseudomonas,[28] and *Mycobacterium avium* complex (MAC).[29]

APPLICATIONS. Viola is useful in treating bacterial infections, particularly boils, skin malignancies, and scrofula, which is tuberculosis of the lymph nodes in the neck with an overlying ulceration on the skin.

Marrow-Strengthening Herbs

These herbs are important to tonify and vitalize—that is, circulate and regulate—the Xue and Kidney System.

Millettia *(ji xue teng)*

Millettia reticulata vitalizes and tonifies the Xue. Milletol is its main active ingredient.[30] Millettia is the main ingredient in Marrow Plus and is used in concentrated form in Enhance and Tremella American Ginseng.

Pregnant women should not use millettia because it can stimulate uterine contractions.

CURRENT RESEARCH. Millettia is effective in managing aplastic anemia and lowered white blood cell counts that result from chemotherapy.[31]

APPLICATIONS. Millettia is useful in treating anemia, and is also used after chemotherapy or radiation to stimulate bone marrow function.

Deer antler *(lu rong)*

Deer antler *(Cornu cervi parvum)* tonifies the Kidneys and fortifies the Yang and is used for Kidney Deficiency symptoms such as fatigue; impotence; frequent, clear, and copious urination; lightheadedness; ringing in the ears; and a soreness in the lower back. It is also use to tonify the Qi and Xue. The main active ingredients are calcium, magnesium, phosphorus, a small amount of estrone, and a substance called pantocrinum.

APPLICATIONS. Deer antler regulates heartbeat and increases blood pressure. Very large doses can have the opposite effect, causing blood pressure to drop. Animal studies on rabbits have also demonstrated that it may increase red and white blood cell counts. Chinese practitioners often use it to stop bleeding sores, ease toxic swellings, and stop uterine bleeding. When combined with dang gui and sheng di huang it is used for treating problems associated with severely deficient Xue and Jing and problems such as aplastic anemia.

Herbs That Protect the Liver

Bupleurum (chai hu)

The root of *Bupleurum chinense* raises Spleen Qi and is useful in countering the symptoms of Spleen and Stomach Deficiency, so common in HIV-related disharmonies. It also helps to even out the flow of Liver Qi and is particularly useful in treating syndromes associated with pain in the rib cage, alternating chills and fever, a bitter taste in the mouth, and vomiting. One of the most common formulas in which bupleurum is the main ingredient is Xiao Yao San (Bupleurum Sedative Powder). It is the primary ingredient in Ease Plus, which we use in drug detoxification and anxiety disorder and is based on the traditional formula Bupleurum and Dragon Bone. It is also used in Bu Zhong Yi Qi Tang (Central Chi Tea), which is primarily a Qi tonic, to help ease diarrhea and raise Qi. The main chemical ingredients are bupleurumol, saponin, phytosterol, adonitol, angelicin, and various acids.[32]

CURRENT RESEARCH. Bupleurum is important HIV therapy because of its ability to protect the liver from damage and its antibacterial effect against *Mycobacterium tuberculosis*.

APPLICATIONS. Bupleurum is used in formulas for chronic hepatitis as well as for the treatment of CFIDS (chronic fatigue immune dysfunction syndrome).[33] It also reduces fevers associated with upper respiratory infections. In addition, it is an important part of several sedative, anti-anxiety, anti-depression teas.

Eclipta (han lian cao)

Eclipta prostrata's main function is to protect Liver and Kidney Yin. It is also known as a Cool Xue and Stop Bleeding herb. It is the chief ingredient in Eclaptex, the formula most often used in the comprehensive herbal program for people with chronic viral hepatitis. It can be helpful in treating people who have developed sensitivity to environmental pollutants and it protects the liver if it is exposed to harmful chemicals and toxins.

CURRENT RESEARCH. Prof. Dr. Hildebert Wagner, of the Institut für Pharmazeutische Biologic at the University of Munich in Germany, considers Eclipta one of the most promising liver protective compounds.[34] In a Chinese study, when used with supportive therapy, it was found to be effective in treating diphtheria.

APPLICATIONS. Eclipta is used in formulas to protect the liver from everyday chemical damage and to prevent further liver damage as a result of chronic viral hepatitis.

Silybum *(milk thistle)*

Silybum marianum, or milk thistle, is a Western herb that has long been used in Europe for the treatment of liver disorders.[35] Formulas such as Ecliptex, which is milk thistle–based, are effective when used in conjunction with immune-modulating formulas such as Enhance or Tremella American Ginseng because chronic viral hepatitis is thought to be an immune dysfunction disorder as well as a viral disease. The main active ingredients are silymarin and flavolignans.[36]

CURRENT RESEARCH. Silybum has been shown to stimulate liver cell proteins, leading to more rapid recovery of liver cells after they have been damaged.[37]

APPLICATIONS. Silybum is a part of formulas designed to protect the liver and formulas that are antioxidants.

8

Controlling the Flow: Acupuncture and Moxibustion

I was in one of the first AZT studies and I had to drop out after 11 weeks because it made me very sick. But that was my springboard to the East. I started seeing an acupuncturist and loved going because it was so nurturing and I could talk about my emotional problems. Now I receive acupuncture regularly and I take herbs for specific problems that arise.

—John, 38, lawyer, diagnosed in 1989

ACUPUNCTURE

When archaeologists excavated the tomb of the Chinese prince of Chungshan in 1968, they found a set of 2,000-year-old, thin, metal probes—four gold and five silver. It seems the monarch didn't want to arrive at the other side without this potent weapon against ill health: acupuncture needles.

Since the prince's day, the needles have become thinner and they are now made of stainless steel, but the principles and practices are much the same as then. The ancient Chinese understood the intricate relationship between manipulating the flow of Qi and other Essential Substances and good health.

How Acupuncture Works

In Traditional Chinese Medicine there are 365 basic acupuncture points (more than 2,500 points have been identified, but the average practitioner uses 150). These points act like gates along an intricate network of channels that transport Essential Substances throughout the body. When specific points along the channels are stimulated using needles or other means, the gates open or shut. The flow of Essential Substances is changed: Excesses are dispersed, deficiencies are quenched. The distribution of Essential Substances throughout the whole system of channels becomes more evenly balanced. This regulatory process harmonizes the mind/body/spirit.

Acupuncture's power to influence psychological as well as physical health was confirmed by a recent study, funded by the National Institutes of Health's Office of Alternative Medicine, that looked at the treatment of 33 seriously depressed women. Among those who received acupuncture, over half experienced complete remission.

What Acupuncture Feels Like

It can prick a bit or tingle and produce localized heaviness and internal warmth. Sometimes it produces a dreamy floating sensation. As muscles relax you may twitch slightly.

The Impact of Acupuncture

Your Chinese medicine practitioner may use acupuncture to create changes in your internal balance in one of six ways:

1. *Tonifying* (or reinforcing) is used when there are no strong pathogenic forces at work in the body. The preventive use of acupuncture bolsters the Organ Systems and replenishes Yin, Yang, Qi, Xue.
2. *Sedating* (or reducing) dispels pathogenic factors such as heat, cold, or dampness and breaks up areas of stagnation. Caution must be exercised when reducing is used in the presence of a deficiency syndrome.
3. *Warming* helps harmonize Essential Substances by removing blockages in the channels. This nourishes Qi, dispels cold, and restores Yang.
4. *Clearing* dispels heat and helps the body reharmonize in the presence of heat-triggered disharmonies.
5. *Ascending* raises Qi, prevents sinking Qi, and prevents Organ System prolapse, such as a fallen bladder or uterus.
6. *Descending* sends Qi upward, moves rebellious Qi downward, and subdues Yang. It's rarely used when a deficiency is present.

How Safe Is Acupuncture?

Those who are HIV-positive do not want to take the chance of being exposed to other strains of the virus or to secondary infections, so clients are sometimes concerned that acupuncture may pose a risk to them. I want to assure you that there is no danger of transmission of infection using acupuncture: Needles are one-time disposables or are thoroughly sterilized in an autoclave. There is virtually no blood, and there are no confirmed cases of transmission of HIV from the millions of acupuncture treatments done in this country.

MOXIBUSTION

Moxibustion is the warming of acupuncture points by placing burning herbs, called moxa, on the protected skin and is often used as an adjunct to acupuncture. But in treating people with HIV infection, I believe that moxibustion is more essential than acupuncture. In fact, I think it is the main therapy and acupuncture is secondary.

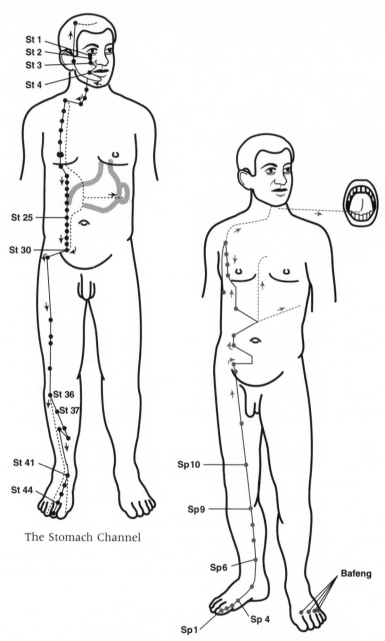

St 1
St 2
St 3
St 4

St 25

St 30

St 36
St 37

St 41

St 44

The Stomach Channel

Sp 10

Sp 9

Sp 6

Sp 1

Sp 4

Bafeng

The Spleen Channel and Bafeng

Figure 3.

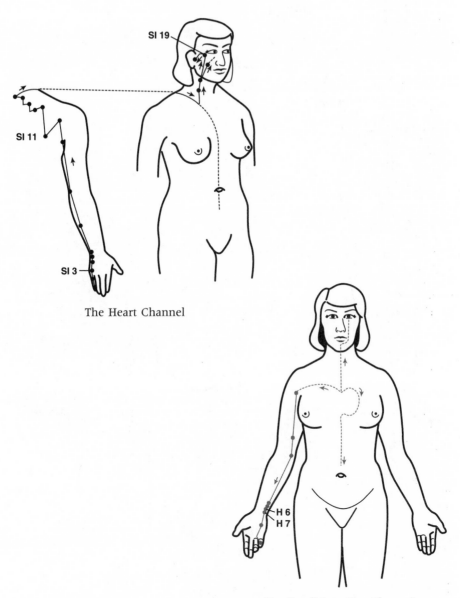

The Heart Channel

The Small Intestine Channel

Figure 4.

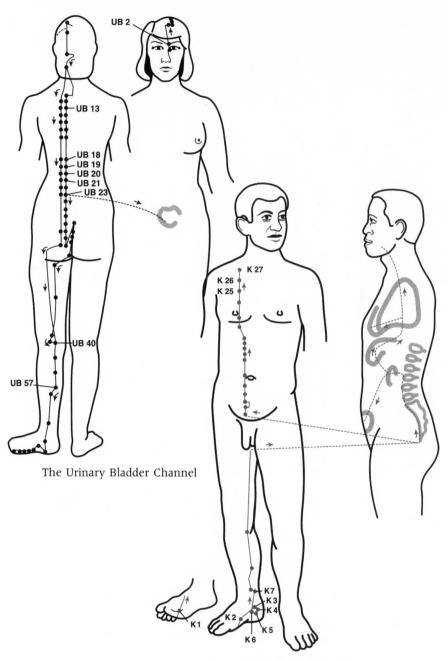

The Urinary Bladder Channel

The Kidney Channel

Figure 5.

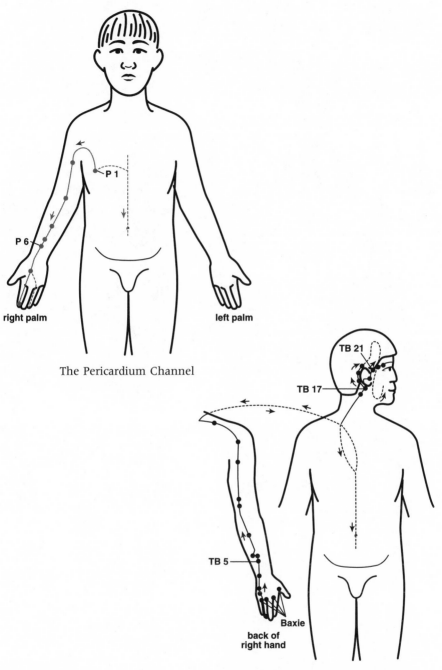

The Pericardium Channel

right palm

left palm

P 1

P 6

TB 21

TB 17

TB 5

Baxie

back of
right hand

The Triple Burner (Sanjiao) Channel
and Baxie

Figure 6.

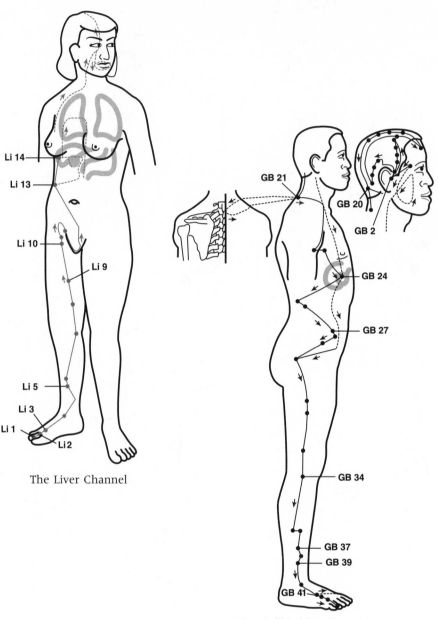

The Liver Channel

The Gallbladder Channel

Figure 7.

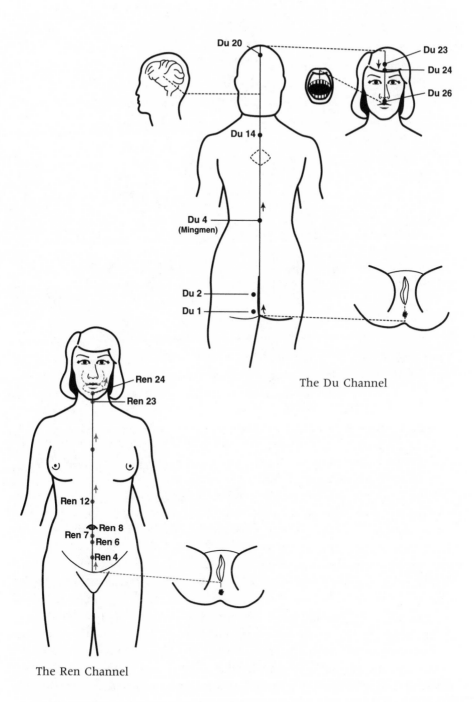

The Du Channel

The Ren Channel

Figure 8.

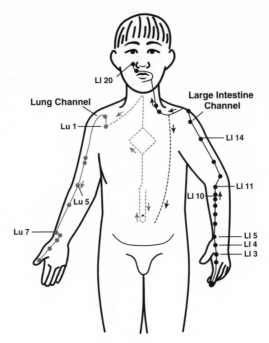

The Lung Channel
The Large Intestine Channel
Figure 9.

This is due to moxibustion's unique ability to help ease the main HIV-related deficiencies of the Spleen, Stomach, and bone marrow. It is also used to dispel cold and dampness and to stimulate the flow of Qi so that Organ Systems are nourished and harmonized.

Early on in my treatment of people with HIV infection, I determined that no matter what else we do in the clinic, we need to use moxibustion on the points Stomach 36 and Spleen 6 for digestion-related conditions and to strengthen Spleen and Stomach, and on Gallbladder 39 to strengthen the marrow. In addition, we use moxibustion on Ren 6 or Ren 8 (Ren is the name of a channel) to warm and tonify Qi and the Kidney. We also teach people how to do moxibustion for themselves at home. The only time we don't recommend moxibustion is if the person has a severe Excess Heat condition.

At the same time, we always use acupuncture on a spirit point such as the ear point called Shenmen and the point between the eyebrows, Yin Tang.

We are just beginning to understand moxibustion's effects in Western terms: A recent article in the journal *Chinese Acupuncture and Moxibustion* reports that the Nanjing College of Traditional Chinese Medicine found that moxibustion at the points known as Shenque Ren 8 and Zusanli Stomach 36 for ten minutes every other day for two months increased the T cell count in the elderly.

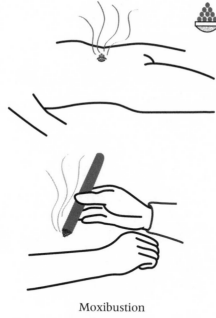

Moxibustion
Figure 10.

Basic Moxibustion Techniques

Moxibustion is done by burning the dried leaves of *Artemisia vulgaris,* commonly called mugwort, on or over the skin. Four methods are commonly used:

• The most common way to use it is to buy the herb rolled in rice paper and shaped like a cigar. This is then lit and moved over specific acupuncture points.

• In the clinic we also place the loose herb in what is known as a moxa box or can, where it is ignited and then the box is placed on top of a protective cloth over the designated acupoint.

• You may put a cone of the herb on a slice of an herb called aconite or a thick slice of fresh ginger and place this over a mound of salt in your navel.

• During needling some acupuncturists may take a clump of the herb, place it on the top end of the needle, and ignite it, so the heat is conducted down into the inserted tip of the needle. This is only to be done by your practitioner. Do not do this at home.

• Direct moxibustion is done using tiny, rice-size kernels of burning herb directly on the skin. This is only to be done by your practitioner. Do not do this at home.

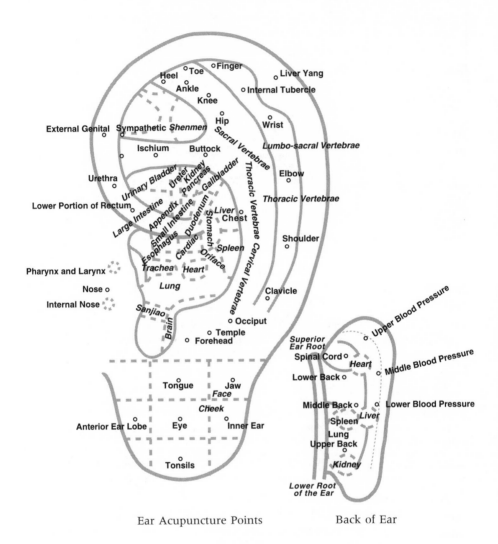

Ear Acupuncture Points   Back of Ear

Figure 11.

CAUTION ON USE OF MOXIBUSTION

Do not moxa in bed, if you are sleepy, or have dementia—ask a friend to assist you. Avoid moxibustion if you have a fever, numbness, or neuropathy. Pregnant women are advised to avoid moxibustion on the torso or lower back.

Self-moxibustion

At home you can do self-moxibustion safely and effectively using a wand or a mound of herbs if you follow these instructions.

Moxa sticks can be purchased in prerolled cigar-shaped wands at the herbalist or from your practitioner. When lit, you use them by circling the hot end of the stick about one inch above the skin, over the designated acupoint. If it feels too hot, move it another half inch away from the skin. Use it until you feel the area is infused with Qi and you are relaxed.

I use the wand in the clinic and prescribe it for home use for clients who are troubled with chronic abdominal pain and painful joints, dysmenorrhea, hernias, and abdominal pain. At home you should mark the acupoint with a small dot or a circle before you begin so you can keep the heat focused on the proper spot.

TIP

Put out a burning moxa stick by wrapping it in aluminum foil or putting it in a sealed fireproof container, such as a lidded glass jar. Dampening it with water or stubbing it out ruins the moxa stick.

Moxa cones are a bit more complicated to use, but you may want to use them for treating chronic diarrhea, using your navel as the "acupoint." The moxa cone is made by compressing the herb mixture, known as moxa wool, into a cone about the size of the upper part of your thumb. The cone is then placed on a round of the herb aconite. (It may be toxic if ingested, so don't leave it around where pets and children can get into it.) You can substitute a 1/8-inch-thick slice of fresh ginger that you have pierced with about four or five small holes. Beware, ginger has a higher water content and sweats more than aconite; it isn't good as insulation and you can burn your skin if you're not careful. The aconite-moxa combination is then placed on the targeted treatment point. The most popular application is to put the aconite-moxa combination on top of a mound of salt poured into your navel. To do belly-button moxibustion at home, follow these steps:

1. Make three cone-shaped mounds of mugwort about an inch high.

2. Place each one on a slice of dry aconite or ginger and put it within easy reach so you can retrieve them while you're lying down without having to sit up at all. You'll see why this is important in Step 5.

3. Recline on a firm, comfortable surface—an exercise mat on the floor is a good choice.

4. Put some clean, flattened cotton balls or gauze and a small towel within your reach, in case you should need it to provide some extra protection during the treatment. Make sure you don't ignite the cotton ball or gauze!

5. Put two tablespoons of salt in your navel and pat it down so it's flat. (If you are an "outtie," the Chinese texts suggest taking a long, wet noodle and forming a circle around the navel to contain the salt.)

6. Pick up one unit of aconite with the moxa cone on top. Light the herb, not the aconite. If you set the moxa on fire from the top it will burn more slowly and produce less heat; burning from the bottom intensifies the experience.

7. Place the aconite with the moxa on top of it over the salt. (If at any time it gets too hot for your skin, you can gently pick up the aconite and slip that towel under it, on top of the salt.)

8. When the moxa burns down, replace the aconite-moxa package with the next one you prepared. When you are done with all three of them, save the aconite and brush the salt off your belly.

9. If you want to moxa acupuncture points elsewhere on your body, you substitute a cotton cloth for the salt and top it with the aconite or ginger.

MOXIBUSTION ON SPECIFIC ACUPUNCTURE POINTS

• *Stomach 36*—Located four fingers' width below the knee, near the bone on the outer side of the leg. This is a major Qi point on the body and tonifies and regulates Qi, harmonizes the Stomach and the Spleen Systems, and is good for digestive disorders and lack of energy. (See page 96.)

• *Spleen 6*—Located four fingers' width above the bone that sticks out of the inner ankle. Known as the Three Yin meeting point, it tonifies the Spleen, Kidney, and Liver, and is good for gynecological and digestive disorders. (See page 96.)

• *Ren 6*—Located three fingers' width below the navel. Tonifies deficiency; tonifies Qi; strengthens the Kidney; is good for gynecological disorders. (See page 101.)

• *Ren 8*—Located in the navel. Tonifies Yang; warms the abdomen; strengthens Qi; is good for all types of diarrhea and coldness. (See page 101.)

• *Ren 12*—Located halfway between the navel and the tip of the sternum. Dispels dampness and treats digestive problems associated with cold. (See page 101.)

EAR ACUPUNCTURE

Ear acupuncture, or auriculotherapy, is also effective for diagnosis and treatment of HIV-related disharmonies. In this country it has become commonly accepted as an effective way to control addiction withdrawal symptoms (particularly for crack, heroin, and cigarettes) and to counter an addict's cravings during recovery. In addition, ear acupuncture can be used to control acute symptoms such as headaches, nausea, anxiety, and digestive upset or menstrual discomfort. You can learn to use it yourself by applying acupressure in place of needles. To learn how to give yourself an ear-acupressure treatment, see ear chart on page 104 and instructions on page 108.

ACUPRESSURE YOU CAN DO AT HOME

Although you cannot give yourself an acupuncture treatment, you can use the art of acupressure to stimulate the acupoints and help ease disharmonies and strengthen the immune system.

In place of the needles, apply a gentle, firm touch: Using the thick, padded part of your thumb, press firmly and evenly on the area. No poking! You can support the effort by using the rest of your hand for support.

Points to Use for Immune System Regulation

- Stomach 36—Located four fingers' width from the hollow made when the knee is bent (below the kneecap) on the outside of the leg and one finger's width over from the crest of the shinbone.
- Large Intestine 4—Located in the fleshy area between the thumb and forefinger along the forefinger bone that goes from the knuckle to the wrist. *Warning:* Do not use Large Intestine 4 when pregnant.
- Liver 3—Located slightly in front of the point where the bone of the big toe and the second toe meet and form a V.
- Lung 7—Located 1½ inches above the transverse wrist crease on the back of the hand and to the outside, above the large bump on the outside of your wrist.
- Kidney 3—Located on the inside of the ankle in the depression between the tip of the ankle bone and the Achilles tendon.
- Spleen 6—Located four fingers' width above the bone that sticks out of the inner ankle. Known as the Three Yin meeting point, it tonifies the Spleen, Kidney, and Liver and is good for gynecological and digestive disorders. Do not use when pregnant.
- See pages 96–102 for location of the above points.

Ear Acupressure Techniques

1. Ear points are tender to the touch when there is a disharmony in the corresponding part of the body, so you'll know when you've hit the right spot.

2. Using your fingertips, a Q-tip, or a special probe that can be purchased at massage supply stores, press firmly and evenly on the point.

3. Breathe deeply and evenly as you apply pressure. Allow your eyelids to fall half closed so that you are not concentrating on anything around you—only the sensation of the pressure of the ear point.

4. Rotate gently around the point in small motions. Keep pressure firm and even. Keep breathing in evenly.

5. Apply pressure for the count of 10. Release. Reapply.

The following ear points are the ones that I have found are most useful in management of primary HIV-related symptoms and associated problems. (For a complete explanation of all points and their functions see my first book, *The Chinese Way to Healing: Many Paths to Wholeness.*)

- Spleen point—For treatment of diarrhea, chronic indigestion, abdominal distention, functional uterine bleeding.
- Stomach point—For low fever, abdominal distention, loss of appetite.
- Liver point—For Liver Qi Stagnation, breast tenderness, irritability, gas, and fatigue that's better when you move around.
- Large Intestine point—For diarrhea and constipation.
- Small Intestine point—For indigestion and heart palpitations.
- Internal nose point—For allergic rhinitis and sinusitis.
- Shenmen (Spirit Gate) point—In the treatment of addiction withdrawal, this provides sedation, restores peace of mind, relieves pain, and clears heat.
- Sympathetic point—For pain relief and nerve disorders.

9

Grace and Strength:
Qi Gong Practice
for Immune Regulation

Train the muscles and skin externally; train the Qi internally.
—Ancient Qi Gong proverb

Exercise and meditation are essential to keeping your mind/body/spirit strong and agile so you are able to adapt to stress and respond to disharmonies. Countless studies have proved their benefits: Aerobics eases depression, improves cardiovascular health, and strengthens the immune system. Weight training helps reverse HIV-related loss of lean-muscle mass. The practice of Qi Gong, which encompasses both exercise and meditation, replenishes Qi, helps promote longevity, and strengthens the body's ability to resist and handle disharmony. Little wonder that protocols for treatment of people with HIV infection now routinely contain a prescription for regular exercise.

Qi Gong can help you manage HIV infection and related symptoms, particularly (1) loss of lean-muscle mass, (2) shallow respiration that contributes to loss of Protective Qi, (3) stress that triggers additional complications in the digestive system, and (4) cardiovascular disharmonies that may contribute to heart disease and emotional distress.

I agree with the idea that exercise is vitally important, but it is equally important that people with HIV infection not overexercise, which depletes Qi and increases vulnerability to secondary infections and disharmonies. That's why I recommend beginning an exercise program with Qi Gong. It can be incredibly vigorous—the Eastern martial arts are forms of Qi Gong—or extremely gentle, yet all forms provide conditioning for the muscles and the spirit. Furthermore, it can be done by everyone, those who simply don't like to exercise vigorously, and those who find that they don't have the strength for other styles of activity. And perhaps most important, the mental discipline that is an integral part of Qi Gong gives people a feeling of calm control over their bodies, a feeling often lost in the anxiety of living with HIV infection.

UNDERSTANDING QI GONG

Qi Gong is the Chinese system of exercise and meditation that provides a path toward spiritual awareness, physical agility, and mental sharpness. There are two types of Qi Gong, one that is active and strengthens your constitution (it is used for immune stimulation in China) and one that is more meditative and is used to pacify the emotions, harmonize the spirit, and soothe disharmonies. There are literally hundreds of different schools or practices—the most familiar is t'ai chi—and you can try various approaches until you find one that pleases you. While this book cannot provide you with an instruction manual for Qi Gong or other important forms of exercise, I hope it will inspire you to read the more detailed section in *The Chinese Way to Healing: Many Paths to Wholeness* or other suggested titles listed in Appendix 5 and to explore the resources available in your area so you can begin a regular exercise program.

QI GONG EXERCISES AND ADVICE FROM LARRY WONG

Larry Wong has been teaching Qi Gong at Quan Yin for several years and has devoted his life to finding the most effective ways to communicate the art and impact of Qi Gong to others. The following routines are adapted by him from his classes. For information on how to contact Larry Wong and obtain his instructional materials, see his more extensive chapter in my first book, *The Chinese Way to Healing: Many Paths to Wholeness*, and see Appendix 5.

Basic Contemplative Breathing Routine

These exercises circulate Qi throughout the body, replenish depleted Wei (Protective) Qi, and calm the Shen (spirit). They can be used to invigorate or sedate, depending on how they are done and what your intention is.

The Breathing Circle

Sit on the floor with legs crossed in lotus position or cross-legged style. This is important so that Qi does not stagnate in the lower body, but follows the breathing path through the torso and the head.

Inhale through your nose to a count of 4 to 8, depending on what's comfortable. For Buddha's Breath: Inhale, extending your belly as you fill it up with air from the bottom of your lungs upward. For Taoist's Breath: Inhale, contracting your abdomen; exhale, letting your abdomen relax outward. You may practice these two breathing techniques on alternate days.

As you inhale, imagine the air—and your Qi—circulating around your body.

Begin by focusing on your nose as the air passes through your nostrils. Guide the Qi downward from your nose toward a spot in your abdomen about one to two inches below the navel. This is the Dan-Tien, and women should not concentrate on it during their periods. Concentrate on the solar plexus instead.

Exhale through your mouth to a count of up to 10 and concentrate on moving your Qi down the torso around the pelvic region and up around to the lower back. Stop at the tailbone. If you can't exhale slowly in a controlled fashion for that long a count, don't worry. Do what you can. The important thing is to retain a smooth, even, calm exhale.

Inhale and let your mind follow the Qi as it moves up along your back to your shoulders.

Exhale and move the Qi up the back of the head and around the top of your head, returning to the nose.

If you have a hard time focusing on the movement of your Qi in the great cycle, don't worry. It will come with time. The important thing is to enjoy the calming, contemplative process and to become tuned in to your breathing.

General Qi-Moving Exercises

The Peaceful Ocean, or Arm Swing (10 to 15 minutes)
Stand in a relaxed position.

Begin by breathing slowly and evenly. Allow yourself to feel relaxed but alert. Ease your shoulders down; let your arms hang loosely at your sides. Exhale and sag ever so slightly.

Bend your knees slightly, with toes facing front.

Now begin gently swinging your arms from the shoulders, back and forth. Let your hips sway gently, too.

As you swing, feel how the motion comes up from your waist—through your torso and into your arms.

Now swing your arms side to side in front of you and begin to twist from your waist as though your torso were a damp cloth and you wanted to wring it out. (Be careful not to twist your knees or ankles—you don't want to put strain on the joints.)

You may alternate swinging from side to side and front to back as you like. Don't think about anything; let your mind clear. Continue the motion for a total of five minutes. When you are done stand quietly and breathe evenly and calmly. When you feel "settled" you may continue.

The Rubber Band (1 to 3 minutes)
Stand with your toes facing forward and your feet placed in line with your shoulders. Begin bouncing gently, keeping your knees bent. Allow your arms to hang limply at your sides. Keep your shoulders relaxed but don't let them slump forward. As you bounce you should feel like a car idling quietly in

neutral. Continue bouncing, arms flopping, shoulders relaxed, for several minutes. When you're done, stand tall slowly, breathing evenly. Relax.

Doing the Peaceful Ocean and the Rubber Band together tonifies the Organ Systems and promotes long life.

Qi Gong Exercises to Build Lean-Muscle Mass

Qi Gong doesn't make you bulk up as a workout with free weights does, but it can provide a concentrated, nonstressful routine for building solid muscle power. In addition, it helps ease digestive problems and strengthens the Spleen and Stomach by keeping Qi flowing gracefully throughout the body.

For detailed information on strength-building Qi Gong exercises consult the books recommended in Appendix 5 or contact Larry Wong to order his instructional tapes and, in the San Francisco area, to take his classes.

Qi Meditation

I use this meditation with clients at Chicken Soup Chinese Medicine clinic to move Qi through the channels, refreshing the entire body and the spirit. It is designed to be done in one sitting, but you may adopt it to use for moving Qi in specific areas of your body if you feel you need a targeted—and faster—fix.

Before you get started, I want to give those of you who have never meditated before a few suggestions:

You may want to record the meditation on tape and play it back while you meditate so that you can follow the steps without having to worry about what you're supposed to do next. Or you may ask someone to read it slowly and softly to you. Once you are familiar with the routine you can do it in silence.

Find a comfortable position to meditate: Sit with your back against a wall or in a comfortable but firm chair if you need support; lie down on a mat; or sit cross-legged.

Qi Meditation Routine

1. Sit in a chair, sit cross-legged on the floor, or lie down.

2. Close your eyes. Close your mouth and place the tip of your tongue against the roof of your mouth. This connects the Yin and Yang channels and allows for Qi flow.

3. With your eyes closed, bring your attention to the area around and below your navel, where Qi is stored.

4. Allow yourself to begin to breathe into the area. You may use either the Buddha's Breath or Taoist's Breath breathing technique. (See page 110.)

5. As you breathe into the abdomen, notice an ever-expanding warmth in the center of your abdomen.

6. Notice the energy moving into the area of your heart and opening into your chest.

7. Now notice as Qi moves to the area below your shoulder blade and then down the outside of your arm into your thumb.

8. When it gets to the tip of the thumb, move your focus to the index finger. Feel the Qi as it moves from your index finger up the outside of your arm into the side of your neck and then out onto your face beside your nose. Breathe in and out as it rests there for a couple of seconds.

9. Then move it slowly to a spot under your eye. Feel it as it streams downward over your face and onto the front of your neck, heading over the front of your torso, down alongside the navel, and around the pelvic area until it comes to the outside of the thigh.

10. From there it should move into an area just below the knee and the Qi should feel particularly strong. From there it moves down the shin to the front of the foot and the top of the toes.

11. Spend time feeling the Qi in your toes. Begin along the inside of the big toe, along the arch, in front of the ankle bone, up along the inside of your leg and the front of your body, around the ribs, coming to rest along the outside of your ribs.

12. Now move your attention up to your heart. Feel how the Qi flows from there toward your armpit, down the inside of your arm. Bring it back up along the outside of the arm, across your collarbone, and up the back of your neck to the front of your ear. Breathe slowly and peacefully for about 30 seconds.

13. Begin again finding Qi as it moves from the inside corner of your eye, up across the top of your head, and down the back of your neck. At that point, you will feel the Qi divide and follow two parallel courses along either side of the spine. These separate routes reunify at the buttocks and Qi then moves down the back of the leg, around the ankle bone, and into the little toe.

14. From there, Qi moves up from the foot, up the inside of the leg and around the navel.

15. Now move the Qi up the torso to the front of the arm and then down the middle of the arm into the palm of the hand. Feel it travel into the fingers.

16. Move your attention to your fourth finger and feel the flow move over the top of the hand, around the elbow, over the shoulder, up along the neck, around the ear.

17. From there it zigzags over the head and comes down the back of the neck, across the shoulder, down the side of the body, zigzagging again on the side of the body, and all the way down over the hip and the deepest point in the muscle of the body in the buttocks, then moving down the side of the leg, all the way down to the top of the toes, to the fourth toe.

18. Move your attention to the flow of Qi through the big toe, out across the top of the foot, and up the middle of the leg until it goes by the genitals and up into the lungs.

19. This is the whole cycle of Qi through the channels. Rest easily, breathing slowly and enjoying the infusion of energy and peace that you feel.

ADDITIONAL FORMS OF EXERCISE

The benefits of exercise are substantial. But the dangers are real as well, as demonstrated in a study at the Naval Medical Center in San Diego that looked at the decline in CD4+ cell counts over time among a group of men who were HIV-positive and were taking various Western HIV-therapies. They evaluated nonexercisers; weight trainers who worked out three times a week and did not do aerobics; and runners who ran three times a week, doing at least eight-minute miles and no weight training.

The reported decline in CD4+ cell counts over two years was 2.1 percent in the weight lifters; 2.7 percent in nonexercisers; and 6.4 percent in the runners. The study coincides with the Chinese medicine perspective that heavy aerobic workouts can drain Qi and lower disease resistance.

Weight Training

Weight training is highly recommended for people with HIV infection when done in a carefully supervised program that doesn't tire the body or deplete Qi. In some instances it is done in conjunction with the administration of Human Growth Hormone or anabolic steroids to build muscle bulk.

Weight training that taxes your muscles to 60 to 80 percent of their capacity helps build muscle fiber and promotes protein retention. This can be done on weight machines or with free weights. To bring your muscle exertion up to 60 to 80 percent of capacity you can increase the weight you are lifting, increase the number of repetitions you do, or increase the speed with which you contract your muscles. Maximum bulking occurs when you increase the weight and/or the resistance.

There is no one weight-training program that you should follow—each person should create a routine tailored to his or her specific body type, physical condition, and degree of previous experience. It is best to start out with lighter weights, doing more repetitions, until you build your strength. You should be able to do about 12 reps of each exercise—if you can't, reduce the weight. Once you can comfortably do 12 reps it's time to increase the weight slightly.

Aerobic-Endurance Conditioning

Aerobic-endurance conditioning is also important for people living with HIV infection. Although there is evidence that overexertion can have negative consequences, moderate exercise routines provide important benefits: keeping Qi moving, helping increase the supply of Wei (Protective) Qi, building overall endurance, promoting good sleep, helping maintain cardiovascular health, and regulating digestive processes.

In a basic routine, about a quarter of the total time should be spent on warm-up and stretching, half the time to the most vigorous part of the activity, and another quarter of the time to cooling down and stretching afterward. You can begin a 40-minute routine with walking for 20 minutes every other day (that means you'll stretch for 10 minutes, walk for 20, and cool down for 10)—or if you are already doing regular aerobics you may follow your usual routine, if it is not too exhausting. You must tune in to your body day to day to judge what is best for you. And keep in touch with your doctor or practitioner to make sure you are not damaging your overall health.

10

Complementing Chinese Medicine: Healing Techniques That Support the Basic Program

In addition to the classical Chinese Medicine therapies of acupuncture, herbs, diet, and Qi Gong, there are several other healing arts that are an essential part of the Chicken Soup Chinese Medicine program for people with HIV infection. Many of these Eastern and Western techniques are detailed in the specific treatment programs in Part IV of this book, and a more extensive exploration is available in *The Chinese Way to Healing: Many Paths to Wholeness.* But the basics of self-massage and of cleansing baths and soaks are set out in this chapter because they reduce stress, and that helps bolster immune strength, decrease depression, increase energy, and soothe the spirit. If you have any questions about whether they are suited to your current treatment plan or condition, ask your Western doctor and/or Chinese practitioner.

CLEANSING BATHS, SOAKS, AND COOL SAUNAS

There are a few basic guidelines about baths, soaks, and saunas for everyone who is HIV-positive.

• Drink two 8-ounce glasses of filtered water or green tea before and after the bath or sauna.
• Never take a sauna that is hotter than 102 degrees Fahrenheit. (Brief baths may be somewhat hotter.) And limit all baths and saunas to 20 minutes or less. Avoid overheating because excess sweating depletes Wei (Protective) Qi, which can leave you vulnerable to Pernicious Influences.
• When taking a soak, fill your tub to the top and immerse your whole body except for your face. Make sure that someone else in the house knows you are in the tub so they can check up on you from time to time.
• In a sauna you can enjoy some inhalation therapy by adding herbs to the hot coals. Soak herbs in water for several minutes before laying them over the coals. I recommend sage, eucalyptus, mint, rosemary, and thyme. (In some instances essential oils of these herbs can be used.)

Clorox Bath

This is the most detoxifying soak. Clorox helps remove heavy metals and cleanses the lymph system. (See Jason Serinus's book, *Psychoimmunity and the Healing Process*.) It's also useful for treating fungal infections and athlete's foot. But *do not* use this if you have breaks in the skin or bleeding.

Pour 4 to 8 ounces (½ to 1 cup) of Clorox liquid bleach in a hot bath and soak for 20 to 30 minutes. Shower after bathing. Do this once a week for at least six weeks. Only Clorox brand is recommended.

Tip: Remember to shower off well after the bath and dry yourself thoroughly with a towel that can take the bleach—a white one is a good idea. Take care not to drip bleach on rugs, bedcovers, or clothing.

Epsom Salts Bath

Used for detoxification and to ease muscle soreness.

Add one to two pounds of Epsom Salts to a tub of moderately warm water. Soak for 10 to 15 minutes. If you get dizzy, soak less time. Two baths a week are effective.

Chamomile Bath

This is very calming to the spirit.

For 10 minutes, steep one cup of chamomile flowers wrapped loosely in cheesecloth in a moderately hot bath.

Soak for 20 to 30 minutes.

Ginger Bath

This is a stimulating and warming bath.

Grate a cup of ginger into a cheesecloth and make a little bag. Toss the cheesecloth into a hot bath. Let steep for 10 minutes and remove. Soak in the tub for 20 to 30 minutes.

Baking Soda and Sea Salt Bath

Add one pound each of sea salt and baking soda to a hot bath. Soak for 10 to 15 minutes.

Colloidal Oatmeal Bath for Itchy Skin

Using a brand such as Aveeno, prepare your bath following instructions on the box. You'll find this is so soothing and healing to dry, irritated skin that you won't know how you got along without it.

Peppermint or Mint Baths

For cooling the skin. Use only when a practitioner prescribes it.

Steep mint leaves or tea in a kettle or pot of hot water until a strong brew is created. Add to lukewarm bathwater. Soak for 20 minutes.

Yarrow-Mint Hot 'n' Cold Foot Soak
Especially good for stimulating circulation, especially if you have numbness or peripheral neuropathy in your feet. *Warning:* Always test water temperature with your hand before submerging feet that are numb or have decreased feeling.

The hot soak: Using a tub or basin, steep one half cup yarrow in boiled water for 5 to 10 minutes, until water is cool enough to put your feet in, but still quite hot. Soak for 2 minutes. Alternate with . . .

The cool soak: Prepare a basin of peppermint-infused water. Add a handful of ice cubes to make the temperature obviously cool but not frigid. Soak for 2 minutes.

THERAPEUTIC SELF-MASSAGE

Touch is always healing, but when you are faced with a chronic disease such as HIV/AIDS, the health benefits and spiritual rewards of massage and self-massage are particularly strong.

Massage not only puts you in touch with your body in a positive way, which may help reawaken emotions and sensitivities that have been trampled by anxiety or illness, but also gives you one more important technique for acting as your own healer, which is an essential part of strengthening your immune system and bolstering your resistance to disease and spiritual disharmony.

Warning: Avoid massage on any part of your body where the skin is irritated, where there is an infection, swelling, or localized malignancies, or where you've had recent surgery. If you are pregnant, make sure your massage therapist is trained to handle the unique requirements of massage during pregnancy.

Soft Touch for Inner Harmony

Use this massage program to stimulate and regulate the flow of Qi and other Essential Substances. And don't hesitate to select sections of it to target specific areas of the body if you don't have the time or desire to go through the whole routine.

All of the following massages are designed so that you can do them to yourself or have a partner do it for you. Either way, you'll feel great.

Step 1: Qi Gong Inhalation/Exhalation Therapy
The breath infuses you with life, helping to refresh and renew Qi. The steady in and out helps circulate Qi and the other Essential Substances throughout the body. Using discipline and concentration to calm and regulate the breath

can positively change your spirit and strengthen your overall defense against disharmony.

To create these benefits for yourself, refer to the Buddha's Breath routine outlined on page 110 or simply concentrate on your breathing until it becomes slow and rhythmic. Once your breath is steady and calm you can move on to the regular massage techniques.

Step 2: Qi Gong Head Massage

This is particularly useful if you suffer from sinus conditions that are diagnosed as resulting from Dampness, or if Qi and Xue Stagnation in the head triggers headaches and depression.

Therapeutic effects: Stimulates flow of Qi and Xue. Helps clear congested sinuses, eases sinusitis; promotes clear breathing and respiratory problems; eases anxiety, headaches, and depression.

Duration: 5 minutes.

1. Rub the bridge of your nose: Place your index fingers on either side of the bridge and move them in a circular motion going up and out. Repeat five times.

2. Move your fingers up from the bridge of your nose to the center of your forehead.

3. Extend your other fingers so they are on your forehead as well and then move your hands over your eyebrows to your temples. Massage the temples in a circular motion five times.

4. Move your hands up to the top of your head and bring them down over the back of your head to the back of your neck. Rub your neck up and down along the tendons, feeling for knots and tense spots.

5. Bring your fingers up to the joint of your jawbone and rub for the count of 5.

6. Return your fingers to the bridge of your nose. Using your index fingers, retrace the steps you just completed.

7. Stretch your neck by slowly lowering your chin to your chest and counting to five. Breathe in and out all the while. Slowly rotate your head clockwise, resting for a count of 5 with your right ear over your right shoulder, then with your head ever so slightly extended backward, then with your left ear over your left shoulder. Repeat, rotating your head counterclockwise.

Step 3: Torso Massage

For Lung infections such as *Pneumocystis carinii* pneumonia and congestion, grief, and depression. I also recommend torso massage for people diagnosed with Liver Qi Stagnation, Lung Dampness, Spleen Qi Deficiency, and/or Upper and Middle Burner congestion. You may massage yourself or have someone massage you.

Therapeutic effects: This is particularly helpful if you need to clear the lungs because of infections or respiratory distress. It eases the difficult breathing associated with asthma. In addition, it regulates the Zong (Pectoral) Qi, which in turn regulates the relationship between the Heart and Lung. When disturbed, it can trigger depression and grief associated with HIV infection.

Duration: 2 to 3 minutes.

1. With well-oiled hands, rub the palms of your hands up and down the chest from the collarbone to the pubic bone in long smooth strokes. Begin breathing in and out with calm Buddha's Breaths, expanding your belly when you inhale, contracting it when you exhale. Continue this in an easy rhythm while you go through the entire massage.

2. Now move your fingers to the soft area under your armpit along one side of your chest. Rub there with firm, circular motions.

3. Slowly migrate your fingers, still rubbing in a circular motion, from that area to your chest. Move between your ribs toward your breastbone. Press hard enough so that you feel a sensation of your lungs opening up and your upper torso releasing. Repeat several times. Do this from both sides.

4. Finish up by repeating the long stroking motion from the top of your rib cage, along the outside of your ribs to your diaphragm area. Repeat several times, ending up with your fingers under your rib cage softly rubbing your stomach area above your navel.

5. With a partner you can use "percussion" to help break up lung congestion. This can be done by hand, or with a massage tool that consists of a handle with a "cup" on the end. You may purchase it at any massage supply store. To use your hand as a cup, bend your hand so that it forms a little teepee with a pocket of air beneath the palm. Lower it firmly and with short, patting motions against upper chest and the upper back. This should produce a round, ponging sound. If you use a massage tool you will be able to apply the cupping motion to your own back. While you do this, you should focus on your breathing, drawing air in deeply to the very bottom of your lungs and then exhaling slowly, purging all congestion.

Step 4: Belly Massage

Use this to restore balance to the Large and Small Intestine, the Spleen, Stomach, Kidney, Liver, and Gallbladder Systems.

Therapeutic effects: An abdominal massage is particularly useful for chronic diarrhea or if you are suffering from intestinal parasites. I recommend that you use five drops of Cinnamon Essential Oil diluted in one tablespoon canola oil as your massage oil to warm and soothe the belly and intestines. Try to maintain a calm, even Buddha's Breath throughout the routine.

Duration: 4 minutes.

1. Stretch out on your back, with a pillow under your knees. Place some oil on your palms and rub them together.

2. Put your right hand open on your stomach above your navel. Place your left hand on top of the right. (Left-handed? Do the opposite.) Feel the warmth of your hands on your belly and the gentle rise and fall of your abdomen as you breathe.

3. Move your hands over the surface of your abdomen in a clockwise motion 20 to 40 times, until there is a feeling of a warm glow under your hands.

4. Now separate your hands so that each palm covers one side of your lower rib cage, above your belly button, with fingers pointing in toward each other. Massage down over your lower abdomen into your groin area. Repeat five times.

5. Now rub your hip bones with your open palms, following the contour down on to the top of your thigh. Repeat five times.

6. Place your hands, one upon the other, in the original position above your navel. Gently rub your belly with a circular motion. Remember to breathe in and out slowly and to concentrate on your breathing.

Step 5: Move-the-Qi Leg and Foot Massage
Various HIV-related drugs and conditions make it important to maintain good circulation in the legs and feet. I recommend this for those with neuropathy and weakness in the legs.

Therapeutic effects: Helps ease Kaposi's sarcoma–associated lymphatic swelling in the legs and feet and coldness due to poor circulation. Should be used in conjunction with acupuncture or acupressure massage of points known as Kidney 3 (to tonify the Kidney) and Stomach 41 (to ease neuropathy and pain in the feet). For locations of these points see the illustrations on pages 96–102.

Duration: 5 minutes.

1. Select an armless unupholstered chair with a firm but comfortable seat. Sit facing front with your back straight and your legs about four inches apart.

2. Oil your hands well and rub them together to distribute the oil evenly.

3. Place your flat palm on the top of your thigh and place the other hand's palm on top of that hand. Your fingers should be pointing down the thigh to the knee.

4. Rub the top of the thigh, moving your hands from the inner to outer thigh using small circular motions. Then slowly expand the size of the circle until you are rubbing from the top of your thigh to your kneecap. Repeat the progression from small to large circles three times.

3. Next, use the fleshy part of your thumb to press into the center of your thigh from the top of the leg to the knee. When you press in, rotate the thumb around the center point. Repeat as desired.

4. Clasp your kneecap in your hand gently but firmly and massage it.

5. Stretch forward so that your hands extend down your outer calves toward your ankles. Rub smoothly and firmly, with long strokes back and

forth from knee to ankle, covering all parts of your calf and shin. Exert light
pressure moving toward the ankle and firm pressure moving up to the knee.
Repeat three to five times.

Step 6: Foot Massage

The feet may not be the windows to the soul, but they are a main door to the
inner workings of the acupressure channels, and any rubbing or manipulation
of the feet has a big impact on the flow of Essential Substances and on the
channels associated Organ Systems. For an acupressure massage, start with
rubbing Kidney 1, the point directly in the center of each foot right below the
ball. This helps keep the Kidney working harmoniously, which impacts on the
functioning of all the other Organ Systems. You may also target Spleen 4,
Liver 3, and Gallbladder 41 to help harmonize Qi and the Organ Systems. (For
location of these points see pages 96–102.) You also may choose to use Western foot reflexology—see Figures 12 and 13, Foot Reflexology.

Therapeutic effects: Reflexology correlates specific parts of the feet with body
organs and systems.

Duration: 3 to 5 minutes per foot.

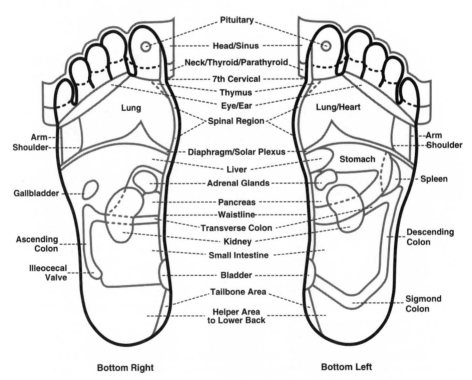

Foot Reflexology

Figure 12.

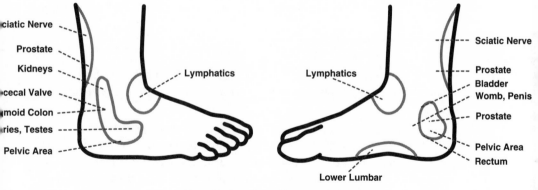

Foot Reflexology Massage 2
Figure 13.

Step 7: Arm and Hand Massage

The hands, like the feet, can be massaged using either Chinese acupoint techniques or reflexology. (See the hand reflexology chart, below.) In either case
you are using a gentle but firm touch to stimulate energy in other parts of the
body.

An arm massage, when done using acupuncture points, can calm the stomach and help ease peripheral numbness.

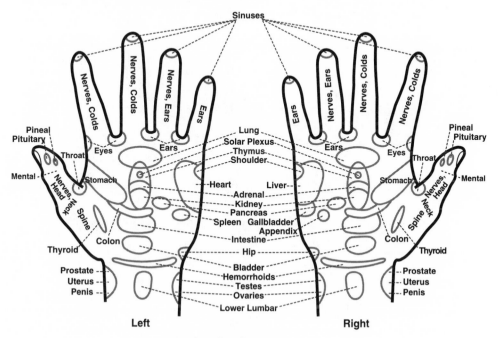

Hand Reflexology Massage
Figure 14.

Therapeutic effects: Particularly good for treating neuropathy and controlling diarrhea.

Duration: 3 minutes per arm.

1. Apply massage oil. Stroke along the arm slowly and firmly from your shoulder to your fingertips. Apply pressure to tissue, not bone. Repeat five times.

2. Next, apply gentle but firm pressure to the points. Large Intestine 14, on the outside of the biceps below the armpit, helps regulate Qi and Xue and ease aching arms and numbness or pain due to drug-induced neuropathy. Large Intestine 10, in the inside of your elbow, helps control diarrhea and regulates the Stomach and Small Intestine Systems. Press slowly and evenly on these points. For location of these points see page 102.

3. Now massage the hands, first the palms, then the back of the hands, using the thumb in a gentle circular motion, pressing on the tissue between the bones and the areas around the knuckles. When you reach the end of the fingers gently pull each finger out from the hand. Shake out your hand. Lie back and relax.

11

Sexual Expression . . . after Diagnosis

When I was first diagnosed, I felt like a walking toxic waste dump. I thought, "That's the end of your life" and "Make sure you don't infect anyone else." But I went to Body Positive support group and seeing normal people who have normal lives and jobs and relationships, that made the difference for me. Today I am in a wonderful relationship with a man who is also HIV-positive. The love is very sustaining.

> —Steve, an M.D. and acupuncturist, diagnosed in 1985

When I found out that my husband infected me with HIV, I was so angry, I can't even describe the rage. It's as though you think your entire being will turn into a red-hot cinder. And at the same time I felt like such an idiot for not knowing that he was sleeping around. I hated him and I hated myself. But eventually you realize you can't live like that—and I was living, year after year. He's dead now and I genuinely feel like I've moved past my anger. You know when I realized that was true—the first time I thought, "Hey, it would be awful nice to have sex with someone again." Then I knew—his poison was gone from my spirit even if his infection lived on in me.

> —Marion, 38, physicist, diagnosed in 1986

Just because you have been diagnosed with HIV disease doesn't mean the end of your sexual feelings or need for physical intimacy. Immediately following diagnosis you may not be interested in sexual expression, but as you begin to live with HIV disease you will probably find your sexual feelings return. In this chapter we will explore the Chinese approach to sexual expression and see how it can enhance the sex life of heterosexual women and men, gay men, lesbians, and transgendered people with HIV disease. If you are working with a Chinese medicine practitioner, he or she should be able to advise you about using traditional sexual practices. Not only are they enjoyable, they are also particularly helpful to someone who is chronically ill and needs to preserve and strengthen both Qi and Jing—the life essence that is depleted through ejaculation and childbirth.

CHINESE MEDICINE AND SEX

Chinese medicine recognizes sex as part of the dynamic life force: The Taoists have long believed that harnessing sexual energy promotes longevity, immortality, and health and that squandering sexual energy leads to depletion, illness, and self-destruction of the mind/body/spirit.

This concept of sexual activity underlies the much-advocated Eastern practice of withholding ejaculation for both men and women during sex. Ejaculation, orgasm, and childbirth are thought to expend Qi—the life force—and Jing—the life essence. For those who are chronically ill, conserving these Essential Substances is particularly important, and Chinese sexual practices offer methods of expression that are highly erotic and satisfying without draining energy needed to maintain health and battle disease.

SEXUAL EXPRESSION FOR PLEASURE AND HEALTH

The foundations of Chinese sexual practices are touch and breathing and meditation. By using Qi Gong exercises and breathing techniques along with various sexual practices you can transform your sexual activity so that it pacifies the Heart System, calms the Shen, regulates the Qi, and conserves Kidney Jing.

EROTIC CHINESE MASSAGE. The rules for an erotic Chinese massage are simple: All parts of the body except the genitals may be touched; stroking should be firm but gentle; and both partners (if there are two of you involved) should be comfortable. I recommend the Qi Gong massage on page 118, which traces the basic route of the channels.

The most provocative points for sexual arousal according to Valentin Chu, author of *The Yin-Yang Butterfly,* are located on a line starting at the navel and going straight down to the genitals. He recommends they be stroked and pressed with the palm of the hand. For women, he also recommends a circle of points around the breasts and nipples; for men, he describes the Mingmen or Life Gate, located immediately below the second lumbar vertebrae, on the backbone a little below the waist, as an erection center.

MEDITATION AND BREATHING. Chinese medicine's use of Qi Gong to help keep sexual energy balanced has been documented since the sixth century B.C. The basic techniques combine breathing and meditation exercises. They are designed to move Qi throughout the body and to calm the mind and spirit so tension and stress do not interfere with inner emotions and drives.

I recommend that you use the Buddha's Breath routine (page 110) every morning and during times of sexual interplay to recycle and repurpose sexual energy. When done actively while aroused, it allows orgasmic energy to be redirected to the inside of the body (instead of released outward) and increases pleasure.

Another powerful routine combines the Buddha's Breath with a medita-

---

HIV/AIDS AND SAFE SEX

Along with a rekindled—and redefined—interest in sexuality and sensuality is the necessary commitment to safer sex—sex that is safe for the person with HIV and safe for the partner, whether HIV-positive or HIV-negative.

No one has done more to spread the word about safe, satisfying sex than River Huston, author of *HIV, Sex and the Single Person.* She gives frequent seminars and lectures to health-care providers, Chinese medicine practitioners, and those who are, as she is, HIV-positive. (For more information on her programs, see Appendix 5.)

RIVER HUSTON'S BASIC GUIDE

Unsafe Sex = unprotected vaginal, anal, or oral sex. Exchange of bodily fluids.

Safer Sex = French kissing, simulated oral sex, genital stimulation, vaginal intercourse with a condom, anal intercourse with a condom.

Safe Sex = abstinence, hugging, full body massage, masturbation, grinding, taking a bath or shower together, using sex toys, kissing, dancing, fantasy, props.

---

tion known as Opening the Flower. This bestows peace of mind and helps you tune into your body in ways that you may not expect. During sexual activity, you and your partner may use this meditation in combination with a Qi Gong erotic massage to heighten sensations and redirect sexual energy inward—deferring ejaculation for both men and women.

- Sit peacefully with your eyes half closed, breathing evenly.
- Feel the air fill up your body. Imagine that you are absorbing your sexual and sensual sensations and drive. Move those feelings with your breath.
- As you inhale, your breath and your sensations move into your nostrils, down through your torso, around the genitals. And see them move up your back to the top of your head and back to the nose as you exhale through your mouth.
- Repeat several times.
- After a few cycles, shift your attention as you breathe in and out to your breastbone. As you inhale feel the air opening up your Heart.
- Now imagine your sexual energy moving up from your perineum (the area between the genitals and the anus), up through your spine, into your brain. Feel your head expand and then as you exhale, move the energy down into your belly, surrounding your navel. Repeat three times. Then sit quietly,

your mind cleared, breathing evenly. You'll find this is extremely sensual when done within a sexual context—but you will never feel drained or depleted.

I hope that you will investigate further the various sexual techniques that are available in Chinese and other traditions and open your heart to the healing joy of sensuality and sexuality. The basic life force—sex—can strengthen the life essence—Jing. And you can have a lot of fun exploring the connection.

PART IV

East/West Models for Taking Charge of Your Own Care

The Basic Comprehensive HIV+ Treatment Program plus 14 Targeted Treatment Plans for Opportunistic Infections and HIV/AIDS-Related Disorders

This section offers the basic comprehensive program for all people who are HIV-positive, plus 14 targeted programs with specific therapies for HIV-related disharmonies and opportunistic infections. All programs combine Chinese, Western, and natural healing therapies, but they do not reflect the full scope of treatment possibilities that are available from your Chinese or Western practitioner. For some of the disharmonies and disorders there are extensive treatment modalities, exploring the use of everything from massage to moxibustion, nutritional supplements to psychostimulants. For others there are simpler approaches, concentrating on a balance of traditional Chinese treatments and targeted Western therapies.

The goal of these diverse programs is to help you create the most effective treatment plans for a wide variety of opportunistic diseases and disorders. You may use them as models for working with your practitioners to create additional plans that meet your individual needs.

THE BASIC COMPREHENSIVE HIV+ TREATMENT PROGRAM

This program is a brief synopsis of the basic dietary, acupuncture, herbal, and Qi Gong treatments outlined in Parts II and III of this book. All the treatment programs that follow offer specific therapeutic guidelines to be used in addition to those in the basic program.

Treatment Options for HIV/AIDS

1. Obtain a Chinese medicine evaluation and diagnosis. You should provide your practitioner with information on all your most recent diagnostic test results, Western medications, supplements, recreational drugs, and activities.

2. Obtain a Western medical diagnosis and evaluation, including tests for viral load and CD4+ count, hepatitis panel, stool tests (if indicated), complete blood count (CBC), and chemistry panels.

3. Share information about the diagnosis and recommended treatments with your Chinese and Western practitioners. If you wish, arrange for them to talk about integrating the treatment process.

Self-care Treatment for People with HIV/AIDS

Diet
Begin a daily journal of your food and drink, along with notes on all medications and recreational drugs (including alcohol and cigarettes), and your range of emotions during the day. After one to two weeks analyze the information and discuss it with both your Chinese and Western practitioner.

Follow the Five-Phase cleansing diet recommendations as they apply to your individual situation. (For more suggestions, see Chapter 6.)

Exercise
Begin Qi Gong exercises to strengthen and balance Qi and Shen. Expand activities to include aerobic and weight-training exercises to help prevent weight loss and build strength. Please consult with your practitioners before beginning any strenuous program. (For suggestions, see Chapter 9.)

Self-massage
The regular use of self-massage, reflexology, and partnered massage at home provides balance and eases anxiety. See the massage section on page 118 and suggested reading in Appendix 5.

Moxibustion

Daily self-moxibustion provides an opportunity to keep energy levels even and to counter symptoms before they become entrenched. Recommended points include Stomach 36, Spleen 6, Ren 6 for deficiency conditions, and Gallbladder 39 and Spleen 6 to tonify the body. (For further information on how to self-moxa, see Chapter 8, page 95.)

Basic Program for Practitioner-Assisted Care for People with HIV/AIDS

Herbs

All herbal preparations should be taken only under the supervision of a trained practitioner or medical doctor, with the exception of the few items listed in Appendix 3.

• The basic herbal pill formulas used at Chicken Soup Chinese Medicine and Quan Yin to treat most people with HIV infection are Enhance, Tremella American Ginseng, and Source Qi.

• For tonification and Clear Heat Clean Toxin (immunoregulating and antiviral) the base formulas are Enhance and Tremella American Ginseng.

• For predominant Stomach/Spleen Deficiency, Toxic Heat, Dampness, Xue Deficiency, and need to tonify the Center: Enhance.

• For predominant Yin Deficiency symptoms such as dry skin, red skin, reddish tongue color, and heat sensations such as flushing: Tremella American Ginseng.

• For predominant Spleen Yang Deficiency with diarrhea or loose stools: Source Qi.

The formulas used as adjuncts to the basic herbal protocol include:

• Clear Heat—To clear heat and remove toxins that are associated with increased viral load and viral or bacterial infections.

• Marrow Plus—To tonify and vitalize the Xue (blood), for drug-related anemia, drug toxicity, and decreased platelets and white and red blood cell counts.

• Source Qi—To tonify Spleen Yang and remove cold and damp and to strengthen digestion; may be used for severe diarrhea with undigested food, parasites, and cryptosporidiosis.

• Woman's Balance—For regulation and tonification of Qi and Xue (blood) and to treat PMS, hormonal imbalances, menstrual cramps, and hepatitis.

• Ecliptex—To regulate Qi and vitalize the Xue (blood); used for chronic hepatitis and impaired liver function.

For additional herb formulas in pill form commonly used in treating specific disharmonies, see Appendix 2.

Acupuncture

Acupuncture treatments are highly individualized, depending on the current diagnosis and symptoms and syndromes that are present. However, the underlying disease process associated with HIV/AIDS does allow for some general recommendations. (For locations of the following points, see pages 96–102.):

- To calm the spirit—Yin Tang.
- To tonify the Kidney—Ren 6.
- To regulate Stomach Qi—Stomach 36.
- To tonify the Spleen and remove Dampness—Spleen 6.
- To ease Yin deficiency and night sweats—Heart 6 and Kidney 7.
- To help ease skin dryness and redness—Large Intestine 11.

Moxibustion

In treating people with HIV infection, I believe that moxibustion is more essential than acupuncture. In fact, I think it is the main therapy and acupuncture is secondary. This is due to moxibustion's unique ability to help ease the main HIV-related deficiencies of the Spleen, Stomach, and bone marrow. It is also used to dispel cold and dampness and to stimulate the flow of Qi so that Organ Systems are nourished and harmonized.

The main points used are Stomach 36 and Spleen 6 for digestion-related conditions and to strengthen Spleen and Stomach, and Gallbladder 39 to strengthen the marrow. In addition, we use moxibustion on Ren 6 or Ren 8 to warm and tonify Qi and the Kidney. For location of the points, see pages 96–102.

Massage

Regular massage by a trained professional is recommended if it is available and is an economically viable choice. Massage based on channel theory such as shiatsu, Qi Gong, and Tui Na provide specific benefits to the mind/body/spirit because they can be tailored to suit your current diagnosis and to treat symptoms. If a professional massage is not a viable option, enjoy self- and at-home massage with your partner.

❦

TARGETED TREATMENT PLANS
FOR OPPORTUNISTIC INFECTIONS AND
HIV/AIDS-RELATED DISORDERS

PROGRAM ONE: NEUROLOGICAL DISORDERS

In Western terms, HIV infection invades the central and peripheral nervous system and causes neurological problems, including neuropathy (numbness, tingling, and sometimes pain in the peripheral nerves), myopathy (muscle atrophy), and dementia. Neuropathy may arise as a result of primary HIV infection or as a reaction to Western pharmacological therapies such as isoniazid for tuberculosis and dapsone for *Pneumocystis carinii* pneumonia and some antiviral medications such as d4T, ddC, and AZT.

Neurological problems can also arise as a result of HIV-related diseases and disorders such as CMV (cytomegalovirus, a viral infection that often causes blurry vision leading to blindness, difficulty swallowing, colitis, and, in rare cases, pneumonia) and toxoplasmosis (a protozoal infection that causes paralysis, mental confusion, headaches, and seizures).

Combining East and West

The three comprehensive neurological treatment programs offered here are for neuropathy, fibromyalgia, and dementia. If you are interested in following through on them, it is important that you receive a clear baseline diagnosis from your Western physician and give it to your Chinese practitioner. In addition, you should let both practitioners know the full range of therapies you are using. This allows you to shape your care program most effectively. For example, if you are experiencing peripheral numbness associated with AZT, your Western doctor may agree to have you stay on the medication while you treat the problem with Chinese medicine. This would allow you to continue your antiviral regime without interruption, if that's your choice.

NEUROPATHY

Neuropathy causes a loss of feeling, numbness, or tingling in the hands and feet and is generally progressive, leading to severe nerve pain or debilitating numbness. It develops as a result of primary HIV infection, of associated disorders, or of the negative side effects of chemotherapy for Kaposi's sarcoma, AZT or other antiviral drugs, and some drugs used to treat opportunistic infections. Both Chinese and Western practitioners would like to be able to reverse the neuropathy, but that is often difficult to accomplish, and as a result the main goal of treatment is often pain control. Overall, Chinese therapy is generally more effective and less intrusive than Western treatment in remedying neuropathy associated with antiviral drugs and primary HIV infection. However, researchers from the Roxane Pain Institute in Columbus, Ohio, are finding that nonpharmacological therapies such as hypnosis, biofeedback, electrical stimulation, acupuncture, local nerve blocks, and individual and group psychotherapy are effective. In fact, they report that patients who are HIV-positive who receive pharmacological pain remedies say that although the intensity of the sensation is lowered, they do not experience improvement in their levels of distress or disability. Those improvements—so instrumental in management of chronic conditions and pain—come from the alternative therapies that address the mind and spirit as well as the body and give the person with HIV infection some control over management of the pain.

This is another example of Eastern and Western medicine moving closer together because of the common interest in solving the problems associated with HIV/AIDS.

Treatment Options for Neuropathy

The first step is to have a thorough examination by a Western and a Chinese medicine doctor to determine the diagnosis. Then you can begin to plan your self-care routine and explore the treatment options available through your doctor and practitioner.

1. Obtain a Chinese medicine diagnosis. Neuropathy is generally diagnosed as one of five syndromes:

- Damp in the channels
- Deficient Qi and Xue
- Stagnant Xue
- Cold stagnation
- Heat or Damp Heat

2. Have a Western baseline evaluation and diagnosis to determine whether neuropathy is a reaction to medication, a symptom of another underlying disorder, or a symptom of primary HIV infection. Then the Western doctor can recommend a variety of treatment options, including changing medication, practicing mental pain-control techniques, or, in severe cases, even surgery.

3. Make sure that the Western and Chinese practitioners know about one another's diagnosis and treatment. Coordinate their therapies. Arrange for them to discuss your case if you feel it's appropriate.

Self-care Treatments for Neuropathy

Herbal Hot Packs

You may buy or make your own herbal hot packs. If you make them at home, take one loose cup each of fresh rosemary, thyme, and mint and wrap in cheesecloth. Secure the ends. Soak the herbal package in a basin of boiling-hot water. Remove from water and wrap in thick towel. Place towel on the floor on top of a plastic sheet (or garbage bag). Place your bare feet on top of the towel and then place another plastic sheet over your feet to seal in the warmth. Remain until the towel cools. Then it's time for a foot massage (see page 122).

You may adapt this to the hands and fingers.

For facial neuropathy you may gently steam your face with warm water infused with the herbs.

Nonpharmacological Pain-Control Techniques

These include meditation, the practice of mindfulness, biofeedback, self-hypnosis, deep relaxation, and imagery.

The breathing techniques outlined on page 110 offer a good starting point for meditation and mindfulness—the practice of being in the moment and quieting the mind so that it does not amplify the pain.

Exercise

Focus on exercise to increase circulation in the affected areas.

See the Qi Gong arm swing on page 111 for neuropathy in the hands; the Rubber Band on page 111 helps stimulate the flow of Qi in the legs and feet.

In addition, you may use low-impact or slow-paced aerobics and stretching exercises under the supervision of an exercise physiologist or medical practitioner.

Diet

Follow the basic diet program outlined in Chapter 6. In addition, if you are suffering from cold hands and feet, I recommend that you eat lamb and/or ginger congee three times a week (see pages 69 and 70).

You may also want to have half a cup of chicken soup (page 71) daily for one week, then once a week.

Moxibustion

Moxibustion is an important therapy for treating peripheral neuropathy, but you must exercise particular caution: You may not be able to feel when you are overheating or even burning your skin. Therefore, I recommend that if you do it at home, always have a partner there to supervise or apply the moxa.

Once a day with a moxa stick (see pages 95 and 102–106) apply moxa to Spleen 4, 6, 9, and 10 and over the areas of numbness and pain if there is no burning sensation or redness already present. Ask your practitioner before doing moxibustion to make sure you target the appropriate points for the length of time suited to your diagnosis.

Self-massage or Partnered Massage

You or your partner may massage areas that are numb or painful, using long, smooth strokes. You may also use Qi Gong massage for arms and hands and for legs and feet (pages 121–24).

Do not massage areas of the body that are hot to the touch.

If your diagnosis indicates dampness, cold, and deficiency, massage with warming and stimulating oils infused with cinnamon essential oil or Traumeel.

Amber Cream from Spring Wind Herbs is highly recommended by Sharon Hennessey, L.Ac., at Quan Yin.

Practitioner-Assisted Care for Neuropathy

Herbs

All herbal preparations should be taken only under the supervision of a trained practitioner or medical doctor, with the exception of those few items listed in the Medicine Cabinet in Appendix 3.

- For damp in the channels—Formulas such as Mobility 3, particularly for treating the lower body and joints; Mobility 2 when inflammation is present; Ac-Q for aching pain; Cir-Q to warm and regulate Qi.
- For deficient Qi and Xue—Formulas such as Women's Precious Pills (Eight Precious Pill); Marrow Plus; and Channel Flow.
- For stagnant Xue—Channel Flow.
- For stagnant Cold—Channel Flow.
- For Heat or Damp Heat—Clear Heat or Coptis Purge Fire or Long Dan Xie Gan Wan.

Acupuncture

Receive acupuncture and/or electro-acupuncture as appropriate for Chinese medicine diagnosis and to ease pain.

- For damp in the channels—Spleen 6, Spleen 9.
- For deficient Qi and Xue—Stomach 36, Spleen 6, Kidney 3, Spleen 4.
- For stagnant Xue—Spleen 10, Large Intestine 11, Spleen 6.
- For stagnant Cold—Ren 6, Kidney 7.
- For Heat or Damp Heat—Liver 2, Liver 5, Large Intestine 11.
- For facial numbness—Large Intestine 4, Stomach 6, Stomach 7, Tai Yang,

Gallbladder 20, Liver 3, local points over area, electro-acupuncture on face.

- For foot pain or numbness—Stomach 41 and 44, Liver 3, Spleen 4, and Bafeng.
- For hand pain or numbness—Large Intestine 4, Triple Burner 5, Baxie, and Small Intestine 3.

Moxibustion

Especially good over areas of numbness and pain as well as appropriate points.

Moxibustion on same points as listed in acupuncture above—unless diagnosis is for neuropathy associated with heat or Damp Heat. Then moxa is not recommended.

Massage

Professional massage therapy can provide profound relief from both the sensations and anxiety associated with neuropathy. Qi Gong massage that moves Qi and rebalances the channels is extremely effective. Alternative healing massage such as shiatsu, reiki, and cranio-sacral are also recommended. Make sure your massage therapist has experience dealing with peripheral neuropathy, which requires understanding of the unique physical conditions of this syndrome.

Pharmacological Pain-Control Techniques

Western doctors often prescribe nonsteroidal pain relievers and narcotics such as codeine and morphine. These medications should be taken on a regular schedule but it is necessary to monitor yourself for side effects such as constipation, fatigue, nausea, dry mouth, and fuzzy thinking. If the side effects are troubling to you, investigate alternative medications.

Supplements

No vitamins or other supplements should be taken without first discussing the proposed regime with your Western doctor and Chinese medicine practitioners.

- The Quan Yin recommendations (developed by Sharon Hennessey, L.Ac.) for supplementation include B-vitamin complex containing, specifically, biotin (10–15 mg), B-6, B-12 and folic acid, thiamine (100 mg) and inositol (2–6 grains). She also recommends gamma-linoleic acid (GLA), magnesium, calcium, alpha-lipoic acid, vitamin D, and phosphatidylcholine.
- Injections of B-12, available from a physician only, often prove helpful.

FIBROMYALGIA

Another pain-related disorder, fibromyalgia, causes a generalized muscle pain. This often crippling disease of undetermined origin—most likely viral—affects many people who are suffering with chronic fatigue immune dysfunction syndrome (CFIDS) and those with HIV/AIDS. The disorder is often overlooked, or lost in the mix of other HIV-related symptoms. If you have chronic, undiagnosed muscle pain accompanied by fatigue and depression, I urge you to discuss the various remedies suggested below with your practitioner and Western doctor. This is not a full program, but these treatments can help alleviate the pain.

Herbs

Channel Flow is an herbal formula that is designed to work specifically on fibromyalgia and abdominal pain. For pain without heat or redness, your practitioner may prescribe ginger tablets or capsules.

Acupuncture and Moxibustion

Acupuncture eases pain when used in areas of discomfort and on Pericardium 6; Small Intestine 11, particularly for upper-back and shoulder problems; Gallbladder 34, for tendons, muscle pain, and tightness; Large Intestine 4, for pain in head and abdomen; Liver 3, to relieve Liver Qi Stagnation.

Moxibustion can be applied to any area where there is pain without inflammation or redness.

Ear acupuncture: Ear Sympathetic, Ear Shenmen, and those specific points on the ear diagram that correspond to the areas of your body that are in pain.

Soaks

Soaks in epsom salts, sea salts, and baking soda (see pages 116 and 117) are sometimes soothing, but keep the water tepid and do not soak for more than 10 minutes.

Exercise and Massage

Beware of overstimulating the body—that can provoke pain. However, a mild full-body massage can be soothing if done very gently using long, smooth strokes. You may self-massage the acupuncture points suggested above, being careful not to overstimulate or irritate the nerves and muscles. (For location of the points, see pages 96–102.)

Avoid intense shiatsu-style massage and vigorous exercise until the body has begun to heal and the pain decreases.

DEMENTIA

HIV/AIDS-related dementia may be associated with HIV infection itself or with various opportunistic infections such as toxoplasmosis, or may arise as a side effect of various drug therapies. Each type of trigger calls for a distinct diagnosis and treatment, but they do produce some similar symptoms: Dementia can lead to a loss of interest and attention to the outside world, an inability to concentrate, and memory loss. In later stages it may be associated with severe motor problems and confusion.

Treatment Options for Dementia

Many people with HIV-related dementia will need the assistance of a partner or caregiver to follow the self-care aspects of this program.

Have both your Chinese and Western physician evaluate your complaints of memory loss, mood swings, forgetfulness, lethargy, etc. They will want to determine whether the mental changes are a result of another associated condition, such as toxoplasmosis, or of the primary disorder.

1. Obtain a Chinese medicine diagnosis. In Chinese medicine there are two main diagnoses associated with dementia: Shen disturbance and Lack of Shen.

When combined with Qi stagnation, Shen disturbance can lead to depression, irritability, and a change of personality. It is associated with forgetfulness, disorientation, insomnia, and lackluster eyes. It also triggers digestive upsets, anxiety, chronic headaches, even psychosis. Any program to ease Shen imbalances focuses on restoring harmonious flow of Qi and Xue and balancing the Heart and Liver Systems.

Lack of Shen is associated with an inability to communicate and a very flat affect—what psychologists characterize as a ''bovine'' effect. This is a very serious disharmony.

2. Obtain a complete Western diagnostic evaluation. For physiologically based mental disorders, Western physicians offer psychostimulants such as dextroamphetamine to improve mood and coordination; for delirium and agitation associated with late-stage AIDS they may use neuroleptic drugs such as haloperidol, although there are potentially unpleasant side effects.

3. Make sure that Western and Chinese practitioners each know about the diagnosis and treatment suggested by the other. Coordinate their therapies. Arrange for them to discuss your case if you feel it's appropriate.

Self-care Treatments for Dementia

In addition to the guidelines in the Basic Comprehensive HIV+ Treatment Program, try the following:

Diet

- Add foods to your diet that can ease deficient Xue such as oysters, liver, and chicken.
- Choose foods that sedate excess Liver such as beef, chicken livers, celery, kelp, mussels, nori, and plums.
- Avoid raw fruit and vegetables, cold liquids or ice, coffee, fried foods, excessively spicy foods, heavy red meat, sugar, and sweets.

Exercise

Qi Gong exercise affects the Shen and spirit directly and almost immediately begins to reharmonize the flow of Qi and Xue. Particularly important are the breathing exercises on page 110. Taking a t'ai chi class is also highly recommended. Aggressive or forceful aerobics or weight lifting generally are not recommended. If you are not suffering from deficient Qi you may progress to 30 minutes a day of more aerobic Qi Gong exercises and then to Western aerobics or weight lifting, which have been shown to ease depression and anxiety. However, go slowly.

Meditation

Use visualizations in which you imagine a beautiful peaceful scene floating on the inside of your eyelid, while doing Buddha's Breath (page 110).

Lie down in a comfortable position with your eyes closed halfway.

Imagine a beautiful environment—the ocean or a meadow or the mountains. Smell the air, feel the sun on your face, hear the sounds of nature.

As you breathe in the beauty let it infuse your spirit. As you exhale, feel the tension leaving your body.

Continue for five minutes—eventually you may work your way up to 20 minutes at a time.

Massage

Self-massage provides an immediate sensation of self-care and tranquillity. But don't hesitate to ask you partner to give you a massage as well. It can be tremendously soothing to mind/body/spirit. The touch should be firm but not jabbing: Press down on each point using steady gentle pressure. Don't poke. Hold for about 10 seconds and then rotate your finger gently around the point for another 10 seconds.

Concentrate on the following acupoints: Liver 3, Pericardium 6, the Si Shen Cong, the four points on the crown of the head, and Yin Tang, between the eyebrows (see pages 96–102 for location points).

Ear massage is also extremely effective: Target the Shenmen, Brain, Heart, Sympathetic, and Liver points. See illustration on page 104 for location of points.

Reflexology massage on the feet and hands (see illustrations on pages 122 and 123), particularly the areas that are aligned with the head, brain, and adrenal points, helps ease anxiety and calms the spirit.

Soaks

Soaks and compresses made from a cloth steeped in hot, herb-infused water move the Qi and raise the spirits through a combination of aromatherapy, the physical effects of the herbs used, and the calming effect of warm water. A chamomile-valerian soak is highly recommended.

Practitioner-Assisted Care for Dementia

Herbs

All herbal preparations should be taken only under the supervision of a trained practitioner or medical doctor, with the exception of those few items listed in the Medicine Cabinet in Appendix 3.

• To calm the Shen, four pill formulas are often used: Calm Spirit blends Eastern herbs and Western supplements; Aspiration nourishes the brain and calms the spirit; Bupleurum and Dragon Bone also dispels dampness and purges heat; and Ease Plus.

• To help overcome disturbed sleep and mental and spiritual symptoms related to hormonal imbalances, which occur in both men and women who are infected with HIV: Schizandra Dreams, Woman's Balance, and Xiao Yao San (Ease Powder).

• To ease depression and improve short-term memory, *Ginkgo biloba* extract has proved beneficial in controlled studies.

Acupuncture

The following points are often used to improve cognitive brain function and ease mental anxiety or confusion: Du 20, Si Shen Cong, the four points on the crown of the head; Small Intestine 3; Urinary Bladder 62; the ear points designated Brain and Sympathetic. Chinese scalp acupuncture may prove useful: It is much like reflexology in that specific areas of the surface of the head are aligned with the brain function in that area.

If your practitioner's diagnosis is dementia associated with wind symptoms such as dizziness or numbness, Liver 2, 3, and Gallbladder 20 are suggested.

Supplements

Vitamins or other supplements should not be taken without first discussing the proposed regime with your Western doctor and Chinese medicine practitioners.

Herbs are often more effective in treating disturbed Shen than are supplements. However, there are several supplements that, when combined with the other elements of the comprehensive program, can offer support for the Shen. Phosphatidyl choline, lecithin, calcium-magnesium, and wheat-grass juice may decrease agitation and insomnia. Melatonin may also be used to overcome insomnia, but should not be taken for more than one to four nights: It's a hormone and no one knows what the long-term side effects are.

Massage

Professional Qi Gong or long-stroke Swedish massage may be useful on a weekly basis. Be wary of those forms of massage that produce strong psychological or spiritual effects such as cranio-sacral massage or shiatsu. They are best when a person has reestablished some degree of calm, and anxiety has decreased.

PROGRAM TWO: PROTOZOAL INFECTIONS

Decreasing immune strength opens the body up to a wide range of opportunistic infections, including those that come from protozoa, single-celled parasitic organisms that can colonize Organ Systems and create havoc. The most common protozoal infections relating to HIV/AIDS are *Pneumocystis carinii* pneumonia, commonly called PCP, toxoplasmosis, and cryptosporidiosis.

PNEUMOCYSTIS CARINII PNEUMONIA (PCP)

PCP affects more than a third of all people with HIV. (The protozoan is often present in those who are not immune-compromised, but the body is able to keep it in check.) Although effective preventive medicine—Bactrim and Septra, forms of trimethoprim-sulfamethoxazole—is available, some people cannot tolerate the side effects, which include skin rashes, nausea, fever, itching, vomiting, and leukopenia. To help people overcome this response, doctors put people on desensitizing regimes that are often successful in helping eliminate negative reactions. Pentamidine mist is also given prophylactically, although it targets only the lungs and is far less effective.

If a person who is HIV-positive contracts PCP, Bactrim and other medications may be effective if therapy is begun early in the course of the disease. Unfortunately, those drugs too have problematic side effects: Pentamidine, which is delivered intravenously, can cause low blood pressure, high blood-glucose levels, low blood cell counts, elevated kidney and liver function tests, and nausea. Dapsone, another drug commonly used in treatment, also may trigger allergic reactions as well as severe anemia, sensitivity to sunlight, neuropathy, and headaches.

Diagnosis for PCP by a Western physician is usually done with a chest X-ray or a bronchoscope and evaluation of a sputum sample. The old rule of thumb was that the body is most vulnerable to PCP when CD4+ counts fall below 200, but many people with higher counts (around 350, for example) also develop the disease. Since it is such a common, and potentially devastating, opportunistic disease, many experts recommend that preventive drug regimes begin well before the CD4+ count hits 200.

Treatment Options for PCP

1. Obtain a Chinese medicine evaluation. Most PCP-related symptoms are associated with one of four diagnoses: Lung Heat; Lung Damp Heat; Lung Qi Deficiency; Lung Yin Deficiency.

Lung Heat associated with HIV may be caused when Toxic Heat penetrates more deeply into the body and disrupts the Lung Organ System. Symptoms may include fever, sweating, cough, shortness of breath, and a rapid, superficial pulse.

Lung Damp Heat, which may be triggered by weakened Spleen and Kidney functions that accompany the early stages of infection by HIV, is associated with a full, high-pitched cough, inflammation in the chest, wheezing, copious phlegm, no thirst, labored breathing—particularly when lying down—and a swollen face.

Lung Qi Deficiency can trigger a hoarse, whispering voice and reluctance to talk, shallow breathing, a weak cough, sweating, a lack of warmth, and thin white phlegm.

Lung Yin Deficiency may result from chronic Kidney Yin Deficiency or if Toxic Heat settles in the Lungs and burns them dry. However, it is also a common side effect of PCP drug therapy—both Bactrim and Dapsone can cause this diagnosis. In these cases, digestive upset may also accompany the deficient Yin symptoms, indicating that the drug therapy is weakening the Spleen. The result is exhaustion, a dry cough, difficulty sleeping, afternoon fevers, night sweats, dry mouth and throat, weak voice, red cheeks, a feverish sensation in the palms, soles, and chest, and sometimes scanty phlegm, streaked with blood.

2. Obtain a Western medical diagnosis. When symptoms arise, PCP is diagnosed through analysis of lung sputum and an X-ray or bronchoscope. This should be done promptly so that drug therapy can begin immediately.

3. Combining therapies provides a balanced approach to healing. Chinese medicine used in conjunction with Western drugs can speed recovery and ease reactions to medication; it should not, however, be used alone.

Self-care Treatments for PCP

Diet

Once your Chinese medicine practitioner has diagnosed your condition, you can follow these guidelines.

TO HELP TREAT QI DEFICIENCY

- Fifteen percent of your calories should come from meat, and each serving should be no more than 3 ounces. Thirty percent of your calories should come from vegetables and 45 percent from grains and legumes. The remaining 10 percent of your calories should come from dairy products.
- Foods that will help balance your energetics and provide the fuel you need include rice or barley broth, garlic, leeks, string beans, eggplant, sunflower seeds, carrots.
- Foods that you should eliminate from your diet while you are battling PCP include all cold and raw foods such as uncooked fruits and salads. Limit intake of vegetable juices.

TO HELP TREAT EXCESS HEAT

- About 30 percent of total calories should come from raw and cooked vegetables; 50 percent, from grains and legumes; and 20 percent, from juices and fruit.
- It is important, however, to avoid frozen or icy foods and to keep the intake of sugar and dairy to a minimum.

TO HELP TREAT FLUID DRYNESS

- Your diet should place an emphasis on dairy products—if you are neither lactose-intolerant nor having symptoms of sinus problems—and most noncitrus fruits, honey, pork, liver congee, tofu, olive oil, peanut oil, sesame oil, walnuts.
- Avoid foods that will only make you drier: raw citrus fruits and vegetables, all cold or chilled foods, caffeine, and alcohol.

Exercise

During acute stages of PCP, when breathing is difficult and fatigue overwhelming, it is best not to exercise; it will further deplete Qi and Yin. However, during recovery, mild breathing exercises such as the one on page 110 can help rebuild lung strength and begin to move Qi throughout the body.

Massage

Concentrate on the following acupoints to ease breathing: Ren 17, Kidney 25, Urinary Bladder 13 (see pages 96–102 for locations of points). In addition, rub the chest with eucalyptus oil or White Flower Oil. You may also massage your chest using a firm tapping with a cupped hand (see page 119).

Steams

Fill a large 2-gallon basin with steaming water and infuse it with 3 to 7 drops of White Flower Oil, eucalyptus oil, or peppermint oil; or with 2 tablespoons of red thyme tied into a cheesecloth bag; or with 2 large cloves of garlic pressed into a fine pulp. Drape a large towel over your head, and the basin. Be careful to keep your face far enough away from the surface of the water to avoid scalding your skin or nose. Inhale deeply for up to 10 minutes at least once a day. Use as frequently as is helpful.

Nebulizer, a vaporizer designed to infuse the air with "medicated" steam, is the ideal way to create a therapeutic garlic steam. It creates a fine mist that you can inhale deeply into your lungs. Ask your practitioner where to buy one and how to use it in your treatment regime. If you want to use this therapy, do not exceed the following recommendations:

- For people with CD4+ counts of 700 or more and no current medical complaints—once a week for 15 minutes.
- For people with CD4+ cell counts of 700 or less—twice a week for 15 minutes.
- For people with CD4+ counts of less than 200—three times a week for 15 minutes.

Practitioner-Assisted Care for PCP

Herbs

All herbal preparations should be taken only under the supervision of a trained practitioner or medical doctor, with the exception of the few items listed in the Medicine Cabinet in Appendix 3.

In addition to the basic program formulas of Enhance, which is particularly effective in reharmonizing deficient Qi, and Tremella American Ginseng, which is effective in countering deficient Yin, Clear Air is often effective for a cough associated with Lung Heat with or without phlegm. Traditionally lung weakness therapy includes formulas with astragalus, schizandra, and deer antler (see Chapter 7 for information on these herbs).

If the symptoms include asthmatic breathing, your practitioner may prescribe the traditional formula Ding Chuan Wan. For a dry cough or one with thin white sputum, use loquat syrup. For a cough with thick green sputum and green or yellowish phlegm, San She Dan is indicated.

Antiprotozoal herbs are well known in China and may also be effective: *Artemisia annua* is used to treat malaria and may also help manage the symptoms of PCP. Ginkgo leaf also may inhibit PCP—Italian researchers found it effectively inhibited the protozoa in vitro and in rats. They suggest it may be useful both to prevent and treat PCP.

Acupuncture

During the early stages of PCP when there are night sweats and Qi and Yin Deficiency, tonify the body using Kidney 7 and Heart 6. In addition, the general points used for all Lung complications are Lung 7, Urinary Bladder 13, and Ren 17.

During the acute stage of disease when Toxic Heat produces fevers and dryness, Large Intestine 4, 11, and Du 14 decrease the heat.

On the spirit side, Lung disorders often create fear and emotional upset. Kidney 24, 25, and 26 are known as spirit points, associated with the Lung and Kidney Systems, and can ease the disquiet.

Additional Treatments for PCP

For therapy for PCP-related symptoms such as fever or symptoms such as nausea that arise as a result of PCP drug therapy, consult the index for specific treatment programs. For example, for rashes see the skin problems section on page 168. For nausea see the digestive program on page 171.

TOXOPLASMOSIS

For those who are HIV-positive, *Toxoplasma gondii*, the protozoan responsible for causing toxoplasmosis, most frequently attacks the brain. This causes a form of toxoplasmosis called toxoplasmic encephalitis. Symptoms include fever, headaches, seizures, changes in consciousness, and neurological abnormalities. Soon after diagnosis with HIV, it's a good idea to have a test for the IgG antibody to *Toxoplasma gondii* to find out if you have a latent infection with the protozoan. Those who test positive and who have a CD4+ count of 100 or less could begin preventive drug therapy with Bactrim or Dapsone and pyrimethamine.

After their patients have contracted full-blown toxo and recovered, many doctors recommend they adopt a lifelong regimen of suppressive drug therapy to avoid a relapse. Taking Bactrim plus pyrimethamine appears to protect against both toxo and PCP.

Treatment Options for Toxoplasmic Encephalitis

1. Obtain a Chinese medicine diagnosis for associated symptoms. The syndromes usually center on deficiencies of Qi and Yin, leading to severe Lack of Shen.

This Shen disharmony produces a kind of flattened affect; people with this disorder are disengaged. It may seem that it takes about 10 to 15 seconds for what's being said to them to register and for them then to respond.

Other syndromes associated with fever and delirium include Toxic Heat, and Liver Yang Rising–type headaches that cause the face to become flushed and hot.

2. Western medical diagnosis and treatment is vital to avoid the serious complications of this disorder. Western drugs should be the first line of treatment and Chinese medicine should be used to support and enhance the therapy.

3. Combining therapies provides a balanced approach to healing. Chinese medicine used in conjunction with Western drugs can speed recovery and ease reactions to medication; it should not, however, be used alone.

Self-care Treatments for Toxoplasmic Encephalitis

Diet
One well-respected school of thought, known as the Five Phases, states that a diet with an excess of pungent foods disturbs the Shen and that the Shen can be rebalanced in part by eating bitter foods. Pungent foods to be avoided include tangy spices, foods with strong smells, and foods that have an aftertaste such as onion or strong cheeses. Bitter foods to be added to the diet include wild greens, capers, bitters extract, and the rind and skin of certain fruits and vegetables, well washed in a dilute Clorox solution.

Exercise
During the acute stage of toxoplasmic encephalitis, when Shen is quite disturbed and the physical body is depleted, exercise is often not possible. But as soon as strength and will return, mild aerobic activities, including walking, cycling, and swimming, should be used to help move the Qi and ease the Shen disturbances. Left unattended, Shen disturbances can become chronic, depression can develop and be increasingly difficult to shake, and mental abilities may become compromised.

Meditation
Qi Gong breathing and meditation can harmonize the Shen and quell anxiety, maintain flow of Qi, and restore harmony to the mind/body/spirit. See suggested meditation on page 112.

Massage

Self-massage of ear points including the Shenmen, Brain, and Sympathetic points can ease agitation and anxiety and help clear the brain. See page 104 for a diagram of ear points.

Practitioner-Assisted Care for Toxoplasmic Encephalitis

In addition to the guidelines in the Basic Comprehensive HIV+ Treatment Program, try the following:

Herbs

All herbal preparations should be taken only under the supervision of a trained practitioner or medical doctor, with the exception of the few items listed in the Medicine Cabinet in Appendix 3.

For deficient Qi and Yin, your practitioner may prescribe the basic regime of Enhance and/or Tremella American Ginseng. *Ginkgo biloba* also may be given to increase brain function, ease dizziness, and help improve cardiovascular function and oxygenation of the blood.

Warning: Avoid over-the-counter Chinese herbal "cerebral tonics" that are specifically for healing the brain and resolving mental disturbances. Many have been found to contain toxic ingredients.

Acupuncture

To improve brain function, your practitioner may choose to needle Du 20, Si Shen Cong, the four points on the crown of the head, Small Intestine 3, and/or Urinary Bladder 62. On the ear, concentrate on the Brain and Sympathetic points. The addition of Chinese scalp acupuncture, not common in this country, may also prove effective in improving mental functioning and concentration. In China it is used for treating paralysis and brain conditions.

Supplements

The basic supplementation routine in Chapter 6 is important. In addition, up to 1,000 milligrams of calcium a day can help harmonize the Liver and Heart and calm the Shen. Although calcium is often taken in combination with magnesium, the latter mineral can move Qi downward. Your practitioner may suggest that you not take it as a supplement if you have deficient Spleen Qi with severe diarrhea—a common condition for people with HIV/AIDS-related conditions.

CRYPTOSPORIDIOSIS

Cryptosporidiosis is another opportunistic infection caused by a protozoan—*cryptosporidium*—and it is associated with HIV and a low CD4+ level. Transmitted through contact with human or animal fecal material and contaminated water, it produces devastating chronic diarrhea that can precipitate severe wasting. Quan Yin recommends that no one who is HIV-positive drink unfiltered tap water. The risk of infection is too high and the consequences too far-reaching. Also avoid the following:

- Diapering children. If you must, wear gloves and wash hands well when finished.
- Changing kitty litters or scooping up dog waste. If you must, wear gloves and wash hands well after contact.
- Contact with stray animals.
- Contact with calves and lambs and locations where they are raised.
- Swimming in lake, stream, or river water.

There is no known preventive medication available and no drug that will protect against recurrence. For treatment Western doctors use a variety of medications that are sporadically effective and often produce their own side effects. Humatin—which may cause nausea, reversible kidney toxicity, and hearing loss—is sometimes useful. You and your Western doctor need to work together to evaluate the best options for you based on possible side effects and drug interactions. *Microsporidium* is a protozoan similar to *cryptosporidium* and produces the same clinical symptoms of severe diarrhea. Several drugs are used to kill off the infection, but none are effective in preventing initial onset or recurrences.

If you have severe diarrhea for more than several days, do not postpone taking action: The sooner you are able to control it the less damage it can do to your constitution and nutritional health. A stool test to identify the protozoa is essential and quick action to halt the diarrhea should be taken. Western medications are recommended, particularly in combination with Chinese therapy. Qingcai Zhang, M.D., a noted AIDS researcher who is an advocate of combining Chinese and Western therapies, believes that there are some herbal formulations used as antiprotozoal enemas that are worth trying. For details see Appendix 4. The newest treatment is made from bovine colostrum (a substance produced along with milk by cows that have just delivered a calf). It is loaded naturally with immunoglobulin antibodies and is engineered in the laboratory to carry antibodies against *cryptosporidium*. Taken orally, it has had promising results in targeting intestinal crypto and stopping diarrhea.

For the basic Chinese medicine treatment for severe diarrhea, see the program on page 171.

PROGRAM THREE: CANDIDIASIS

Candidiasis, also called yeast infection, appears on the mucosal surfaces and the skin, particularly in the mouth, esophagus, intestines, and vagina. When the immune system is weakened, *Candida* can flourish, causing ulcerations, loss of appetite, digestive upset, diarrhea, and other severe discomfort. Over time, if unchecked, candidiasis can virtually shut down the body's digestive system.

Symptoms of candidiasis overgrowth include abdominal distention, gas and bloating, allergic reactions to food and/or environmental elements, diarrhea, esophageal inflammation, vaginal itching, rectal itching, moderate to severe fatigue, depression, mood swings or crying jags, insomnia, nervousness, and anxiety or depression.

Antibiotics may trigger an overgrowth of *Candida albicans,* as can excess intake of sugars and refined grains; some drugs, including steroids such as cortisone and prednisone; and birth control pills or progesterone suppositories. Septra/Bactrim, the medication commonly prescribed for PCP therapy, is linked to difficult-to-treat vaginal yeast infections in women. Currently fluconazole (Diflucan) is the drug used to try to prevent onset, but it is expensive and has often unpleasant side effects.

Treatment Options for Candidiasis

1. Obtain a Chinese medicine diagnosis. There are five syndromes in Chinese medicine that are associated with candidiasis.

- Spleen Qi Deficiency (with dampness) is indicated when the symptoms are intestinal gas, allergic reactions to food, loose stools or constipation, white vaginal discharge and fatigue.
- Spleen Yang Deficiency is indicated when the symptoms are a feeling of cold throughout the body and watery stools.
- Liver Qi Stagnation is the probable trigger of abdominal distention, gas or flatulence, allergic reactions, uncontrollable crying, irregular menses, and depression.
- Liver Heat produces vaginal itching, rectal itching, anxiety, nervousness, esophageal inflammation, and insomnia.
- Damp Heat in the Lower Triple Burner is associated with loose stools, vaginal or rectal itching, vaginal discharge or infection.

2. Obtain a Western medical diagnosis. Chronic mucocutaneous candidiasis is a complex disorder causing infections of the skin, nails, and mucous membranes. It is triggered by the use of antibiotics or results from overall immune suppression. There are currently very accurate blood tests and stool and tissue cultures that are used for the diagnosis and treatment of candidiasis. Western diagnosis is broken down into the following categories:

The infection may manifest itself as chronic and recurrent vaginal yeast infections. Chronic and recurrent yeast infections in women with HIV have been identified as an AIDS diagnosis by the Centers for Disease Control in Atlanta.

Thrush, or oral, candidiasis is another form of chronic or recurrent yeast infection, as is gastrointestinal candidiasis.

A few years ago, lab tests for candidiasis were not particularly accurate. But now, labs such as Great Smokies in North Carolina have reliable tests for candida in the stool. I always use stool tests to confirm my diagnosis because intestinal upsets can be caused by other parasites, bacteria, or organisms and each needs to be identified accurately and treated promptly. In my experience, candidiasis often cannot be treated effectively without simultaneous or even pretreatment for the other intestinal disorders. Candidiasis is often an end result of other disease and needs to be treated at the end of a course of appropriate treatment. Since many of these intestinal disorders are treated with antibiotics, it is often necessary to provide anticandida therapy prophylactically in conjunction with the drugs.

Esophageal candidiasis is an increasingly common AIDS-related disorder, triggered by the use of antibiotics or resulting from overall immune suppression. If symptoms—including persistent heartburn, nausea, and difficulty swallowing—are present, treatment is generally started without confirming diagnostic tests.

Western therapy includes fluconazole (Diflucan), which can trigger nausea and headaches, and clotrimazole (Mycelex), or ketoconazole (Nizoral), all of which may produce negative side effects, including liver toxicity, dizziness, headache, and abdominal pain. It is imperative that people with HIV infection act quickly to quell candidiasis; use of natural and Chinese therapies first is often recommended, since they can be quite effective and are without the negative side effects.

3. Make sure that Western and Chinese practitioners know about the diagnosis and treatment suggested by the other. Coordinate their therapies. Arrange for them to discuss your case if you feel it's appropriate.

Self-care Treatments for Candidiasis

Diet

Diet has an enormous impact on candidiasis. What you eat and the supplements you take can promote or inhibit its growth dramatically. In addition to the guidelines in the Basic Comprehensive HIV+ Treatment Program, follow these guidelines:

FOODS TO ELIMINATE FROM YOUR DIET

- Dairy products—They create dampness in the Spleen, which can lead to congestion and Damp Heat.

- Sugars—Candida feeds on sugars. Often, eliminating sugar from the diet can have a dramatic effect. Excess sugars overstimulate and injure the Spleen, leading to increased dampness and heat. This applies to *all* sugars, whether from fruit, juices, or candy.
- Yeast products, such as breads.
- Alcohol—It produces sugar in the body and can aggravate or stimulate yeast infections.
- Fatty foods—They increase heat and dampness.

FOODS TO ADD TO YOUR DIET

- Miso soup—One cup a day at breakfast of light miso soup. It contains bacteria that can help recolonize the intestines and fight candida directly.
- Broccoli, kale, and cabbage—Eat one of these at least once a day.
- Garlic—Its antifungal properties are particularly potent.
- Lean white fishes and meats—Emphasize these, and reduce the amount of turkey, chicken, and fatty fishes.

Supplements

- Acidophilus—1/4 to 1/2 teaspoon (usually *Lactobacillus acidophilus;* other forms as prescribed by your practitioner) in unchilled water one to three times per day on an empty stomach. This gives the acidophilus a chance to colonize the intestines. Mixing various strains of acidophilus or other bacteria in one supplement will weaken the therapeutic value. If you decide to take more than one form of intestinal bacterium, do so at separate times.
- Vitamin C—Take a minimum of 2,000 milligrams per day up to bowel tolerance, unless you are diagnosed with severe Spleen- and Stomach-related deficiencies such as watery stools.
- Multivitamin and multimineral, both yeast-free.
- Beta-carotene—25,000 IU, unless you are diagnosed with an Excess Heat condition.
- Vitamin E—400 IU dry vitamin E; it has no oils in it and is less heating.
- Caprylic acid—As prescribed by practitioner.
- Grapefruit-seed extract—As prescribed by practitioner.

Self-moxibustion

Moxibustion is highly effective in removing the dampness and helping control candidiasis. Ask your practitioner to assign the points that suit your particular diagnosis. For severe cases you may moxa every other day.

Practitioner-Assisted Care for Candidiasis

In addition to the guidelines in the Basic Comprehensive HIV+ Treatment Program, follow these guidelines.

Herbs

All herbal preparations should be taken only under the supervision of a trained practitioner or medical doctor, with the exception of those few items listed in the Medicine Cabinet in Appendix 3.

People often have to take the herbal formulas for one to three months to get an effect. Using acupuncture, moxibustion, and dietary therapy in conjunction reduces the length of time that people have candidiasis infection. When people use dietary therapy alone it can take 6 to 12 months to eliminate candidiasis.

There are formulas both traditional and contemporary that are highly effective in controlling overgrowth and associated symptoms: Shen Ling Bai Zhu San, Xiao Yao San, Shu Gan Wan, Long Dan Xie Gan Tang, and Phellostatin.

Acupuncture and Moxibustion

Acupuncture and moxibustion are effective in reducing symptoms of candidiasis throughout the body. The following points are to be used for acupuncture and/or moxibustion as indicated.

- For Spleen Qi Deficiency (with Dampness)—Ren 12, Stomach 36, Spleen 6, Spleen 9, Ren 6, Urinary Bladder 20, Large Intestine 10.
- For Spleen Yang Deficiency—Use moxibustion only on Ren 8 or Ren 6, Stomach 36, Spleen 6, Urinary Bladder 20, Du 20.
- For Liver Qi Stagnation—Liver 3, Large Intestine 4, Urinary Bladder 18.
- For Liver Heat—Liver 2, Liver 5, Urinary Bladder 18, Stomach 30.
- For Damp Heat in the Lower Triple Burner—Liver 2, Liver 5, Spleen 9, Ren 2, Stomach 30, Gallbladder 27.

PROGRAM FOUR: MYCOBACTERIAL INFECTIONS

Mycobacterial infections include *Mycobacterium avium* complex (MAC) and *Mycobacterium tuberculosis* (TB). MAC is one of the most common opportunistic diseases, occurring in 30 to 50 percent of all people infected with HIV. It is transmitted through contaminated food and water and possibly soil. To avoid contracting this often debilitating disease, people with HIV/AIDS are advised to avoid showering in hotels, hospitals, or apartment buildings where large boilers or water heaters are used to heat hot water—they are breeding grounds for the *M. avium* bacterium. At home, install water filters on showers and taps, and avoid potting soil and gardening.

Symptoms include persistent fever and night sweats, extreme fatigue, weight loss, chronic diarrhea, anemia, low platelet count, dizziness, weakness, and enlarged lymph nodes, liver, and spleen. The infection can lodge in a specific organ in the body or be disseminated throughout.

The likelihood of developing MAC symptoms increases as CD4+ cell counts fall below 75, and many doctors recommend taking preventive medication when it goes under 100. Among the preventive therapies used, Azithromycin may reduce the incidence of MAC by around 70 percent; Sparfloxacin and rifabutin may reduce incidence by 50 percent; and clofazimine and clarithromycin may reduce the incidence by 70 percent. Many doctors warn against taking a preventive dose, however. If you become drug resistant, you will not be able to use it later as therapy should you develop MAC.

If you do contract the disease, diagnosis is difficult. Usually it is done with a stool test, a blood and sputum culture, and/or a biopsy of the organ tissue. Treatment may begin if there is a positive result from an acid-fast bacillis smear. Although there is not a standard treatment protocol, many practitioners use a combination of oral and intravenous drugs such as Azithromycin, Sparfloxacin, rifabutin, clofazimine, and clarithromycin. The side effects of the medications range from decreasing the effectiveness of antiviral medication to kidney and liver toxicity, skin rash, and discoloration of body fluids, potentially serious vision changes (even blindness), vomiting and diarrhea, itchy dry skin, joint pain, and fever.

Mycobacterium tuberculosis (TB) is similar to MAC but does not trigger chronic watery diarrhea. Screening tests should be done upon diagnosis of HIV infection. All HIV-positive people with a positive TB skin test and anyone who is HIV-positive and has symptoms of TB should have follow-up chest radiography and a clinical evaluation. (People with very suppressed immune systems may have TB but not have a positive response to the skin patch test.) Preventive therapy with isoniazid is usually recommended for any HIV-positive person who had a positive reading on the skin test, even without symptoms. Treatment for active TB includes isoniazid. If you are taking this drug avoid tunafish and Antabuse. Other medications include rifabutin and pyrazinamide. The former is associated with side effects of rash, fever, gastrointestinal distress, and joint pain, and the latter is associated with nausea, vomiting, and liver toxicity.

The Chinese diagnosis for MAC and related TB is primarily Yin Deficiency; with anemia, Xue Deficiency is present. Sometimes what the Chinese call Steaming Bone disease (typical TB) triggers complaints of heat coming from the bones—a common observation of those who are HIV-positive and develop MAC/TB.

There are a few suggestions for specific MAC-related therapies:

• MAC herb formulas include the traditional chin-chiu and tortoise shell. For MAC-related night sweats and afternoon fevers, use Zhi Bai Di Huang Wan.

• Moxibustion should be done at home daily on the lower half of the body only, using recommendations for the lower body from the basic program on page 133. If you have a high fever, do not moxa at all.

• For lung-related problems use acupuncture on Urinary Bladder 13, Lung 7, and Ear Lung.

• Regular acupuncture for sweats includes Heart 6, Kidney 7. For general heat symptoms: Large Intestine 11; Du 14; Large Intestine 4; Lung 5.

• Dietary therapy focuses on adding cooling foods such as apples, bananas, barley, celery, cucumber, eggplant, gluten, lettuce, pears, peppermint, radish, Swiss chard, spinach, soybeans, tangerine, tofu, watercress, wheat, and wheat bran to your daily menus. Cold foods should also be included in your diet, but eaten less frequently: asparagus, clams, crab, kelp, mango, mulberry, mung bean sprouts, nori, octopus, persimmon, plantain, romaine lettuce, salt, seaweed, tomato, watermelon.

The main contribution of Chinese medicine to the management of MAC and related symptoms is through control of severe diarrhea (page 171) and fevers.

PROGRAM FIVE: OPPORTUNISTIC VIRAL INFECTIONS

Many varieties of opportunistic viral infections are associated with HIV infection. They include the *Herpes simplex* and *H. zoster* viruses, which cause oral and genital herpes and shingles; human papilloma virus, which causes genital warts; and the cytomegalovirus (CMV), which can trigger symptoms in the eyes, the gastrointestinal system, and the esophagus. In addition to the basic immune-strengthening herb formulas Enhance and Tremella American Ginseng, some general antiviral herbal formulas are used to attack opportunistic viral infections: Clear Heat contains Clear Heat Clean Toxin herbs for chronic infections, and Isatis Gold formula is useful for acute infections. Isatis-based formulas are used to support Western drug therapy for CMV.

CYTOMEGALOVIRUS (CMV)

CMV is frequently the first AIDS-defining opportunistic infection. A member of the herpes family, this virus is difficult to eradicate completely once contracted and requires lifelong suppressive therapy to control.

If you develop CMV, the symptoms include:

• Retinitis—Blurred vision leading to blindness, retinitis affects more than 45 percent of all people with AIDS. Weekly self-testing using the Amsler Grid can reveal early-stage disease. The Amsler Grid is a 5-x-5-inch square divided into 400 equal-size squares, with a large dot at the center point. If, when focusing on the center point, you notice an area of the lines that are all squiggly or an area where the lines disappear, you should go to the doctor for immediate testing.

• Esophagitis—Pain and difficulty swallowing, ulcerations. Biopsy and endoscopy may be needed to diagnose.

• Colitis—Fever, diarrhea, abdominal pain, wasting. Biopsy and endoscopy may be needed to diagnose.

• Pneumonia (rare)—Fever, dry nonproductive cough, difficulty breathing, weight loss, night sweats, fatigue, and elevated liver enzymes.

Treatment Options for Cytomegalovirus

1. Obtain a Chinese medicine evaluation and diagnosis. Gastrointestinal CMV is associated with Spleen Qi Deficiency and cold conditions. Retinal CMV is associated with Kidney Deficiency and weakness.

2. Obtain a Western medical evaluation and diagnosis. When your CD4+ count hits 100, some of you may want to begin preventive drug therapy using ganciclovir or foscarnet to avoid the serious symptoms of CMV: blindness, wasting, and severe gastrointestinal problems. Consult with your physician; there is some debate about the efficacy of this approach.

Side effects for ganciclovir are reversible and include confusion, disorientation, fever, and rash. Side effects for foscarnet include severe kidney damage, anemia, nausea, low white blood cell counts, and penile ulcerations in uncircumcised men. With continuous creatine serum and electrolyte monitoring, irreversible damage can be prevented.

If you are not on preventive therapy, when CD4+ counts fall below 100, regular testing for CMV is vital to catch the problem early on. Those who are HIV-positive need to be aware that CMV is shed through semen, cervical secretions, and saliva.

3. Make sure that Western and Chinese practitioners know about one another's diagnosis and treatment. Coordinate their therapies. Arrange for them to discuss your case if you feel it's appropriate. It is not appropriate to use Chinese medicine alone for treatment of CMV.

Self-care for Treatment of Cytomegalovirus
In addition to the guidelines in the Basic Comprehensive HIV+ Treatment Program:

Diet
To help the body fight the effects of intestinal or esophageal CMV, such as lack of appetite, loose stools, and fatigue, expand your diet to contain several servings a day of warming foods: squash; carrots and yams; root vegetables such as rutabagas, turnips, leeks, onions; grains such as rice and oats; small amounts of chicken, turkey, mutton, or beef; cooked peaches, cherries, strawberries,

and figs; cardamom, ginger, cinnamon, nutmeg, and black pepper; custards and small amounts of honey, molasses, maple syrup, and sugar.

In addition, eliminate spicy tomato sauces and salsas, citrus fruit, plain or uncooked tofu, buckwheat, milk, cheese, and excess sugar and salt from your daily menus. If gastrointestinal disorders become more severe, leading to deficient Yang, then eliminate raw or chilled foods and all fatty foods.

Practitioner-Assisted Care for Cytomegalovirus

Herbs
All herbal preparations should be taken only under the supervision of a trained practitioner or medical doctor, with the exception of those few items listed in the Medicine Cabinet in Appendix 3.

Herbal therapy for gastrointestinal and digestive disturbances are covered in the diarrhea program (page 171).

For treatment of retinitis, some formulas that include Clear Heat Clean Toxin herbs are useful for countering the negative side effects of the Western drug therapies and for strengthening the visual field. CMV retinitis formula is something that Subhuti Dharmananda first brought to the attention of the HIV treatment community. With some modifications to the original, I have used this successfully in conjunction with Western drug therapy and acupuncture.

Acupuncture
For acupuncture for gastrointestinal complications, see the diarrhea program beginning on page 171.

For retinitis, effective points are Yintang, Yu Yao, Gallbladder 20, Liver 3, Gallbladder 37, and Urinary Bladder 18.

HERPES SIMPLEX AND H. ZOSTER

Herpes simplex (oral, genital, and anal lesions) and *H. zoster* (shingles) are more severe and harder to control in people who are HIV-positive. When they appear they should be treated aggressively, because lesions can become deep ulcerations, and in the mouth or gastrointestinal tract they can interfere with eating and promote wasting.

Treatment Options for *Herpes simplex* and *H. zoster*

1. Obtain a Chinese medicine diagnosis. Diagnoses fall into one of three syndromes: Heat in the channels, Damp Heat in the channels, or Damp Heat with Liver Stagnation.

2. Obtain a Western medical diagnosis; this will allow for immediate use of acyclovir, a potent antiherpes, antiviral drug. Because immune system activity surrounding the presence of an additional virus is thought to stimulate proliferation of HIV, quelling the outbreak quickly is important. Furthermore, use of acyclovir as a preventive therapy for people with frequent or severe herpes outbreaks is often effective. Foscarnet, administered intravenously, can be used in place of acyclovir if infection is with an acyclovir-resistant strain, although foscarnet has severe side effects. There are several newer drugs, such as Famvir, that also offer hope to those with herpes.

3. Make sure that both Western and Chinese practitioners each know about one another's diagnosis and treatment. Coordinate their therapies. Arrange for them to discuss your case if you feel it's appropriate.

Self-care Program for *Herpes simplex* and *H. zoster*

Diet
Follow the general dietary guidelines for the basic program, plus eliminate the following: hot foods such as ginger, cayenne pepper, soybean oil, and trout. Reduce the amount of warm foods you eat: anchovy, basil, bay leaf, black pepper, brown sugar, butter, capers, cherries, chestnuts, chicken, garlic, onions, shrimp, strawberries, and walnuts.

Meditation
The four most important self-care techniques that help prevent outbreaks of herpes are to maintain as stress-free an environment as possible, make sure you get enough sleep, avoid irritating vulnerable areas of the skin, and stay out of the sun. For suggested meditation routines see page 112.

Exercise
Qi Gong exercises will help balance Spleen, Liver, and Kidney Qi. Stick with gentle routines during full-blown breakouts. (For suggested routines see Chapter 9, or read the more extensive section in my previous book.)

For additional information on self-care and herpes, see the programs on dermatological complications of HIV infection (page 168) and fever (page 178).

Practitioner-Assisted Care for Herpes

Herbs
All herbal preparations should be taken only under the supervision of a trained practitioner or medical doctor, with the exception of those few items listed in the Medicine Cabinet in Appendix 3.

Herbal formulas that can help control herpes outbreaks include Clear Heat, Coptis Purge Fire, Isatis 6, Long Dan Xie Gan Wan, Yan Hu Suo Wan, and Liver Fire Rising Formula, a modification of Long Dan Xie Gan Wan formula with raw herbs.

Herbal Salves

Application of topical astringent and antiviral creams can ease symptoms.

Several solutions that your practitioner may provide include vitamin C powder, lysine cream, Sore Throat Powder, Watermelon Frost, and Liu Shen Wan, which is used topically because it contains toad venom and can be poisonous when taken internally.

For *Herpes simplex* and *H. zoster* in early stages when there is tingling on the skin but the lesions have not fully erupted, Dr. Subhuti Dharmananda recommends Gentiana Combination and isatis-based formulas used aggressively in high doses for one to two days.

For full-blown lesions, herbs with tannins and astringent alkaloids are recommended such as coptis and phellodendron.

Acupuncture

FOR ALL HERPES-RELATED OUTBREAKS

- Use Surround the Dragon: needling in a circle around the lesions. This is quite effective.

FOR HERPES ZOSTER—SHINGLES

- Ear acupuncture can be done by your practitioner or you can do ear acupressure at home. Concentrate on Ear Shenmen and Ear Sympathetic (see chart on page 104 and instructions on page 108).
- To ease the pain associated with shingles—Pericardium 6, Large Intestine 4, Liver 3.

FOR HERPES SIMPLEX

- Genital outbreaks—Treat with Liver 5 and 9 and Stomach 30.
- Oral outbreaks—Treat with Large Intestine 4, Stomach 4 and 44, and Ren 23.
- Rectal outbreaks—Treat with Urinary Bladder 57, Du 2, Ba Liao (four points located on the tailbone). (For locations of the points, see pages 96–102.)

PROGRAM SIX: FATIGUE

Fatigue is associated with many aspects of HIV: The primary viral infection itself produces weariness; lack of appetite and wasting are unremitting sources of exhaustion; struggling against all the various opportunistic infections leads to deep tiredness; and fatigue is a common side effect of the powerful medications needed at various stages of the disease progression. In addition, a weakened immune system leaves the body open to assault by the viruses that may be associated with Epstein-Barr syndrome and chronic fatigue immune dysfunction syndrome (CFIDS), two diseases that produce extreme exhaustion.

Treatment Options for Fatigue

1. When you visit a Chinese medicine practitioner you may be delighted to discover that there are effective remedies for countering persistent fatigue. The challenge is in determining the precise diagnosis so the proper treatment can be prescribed. One of the best ways to make a diagnosis is to ask yourself, "Does exercise make my fatigue better or worse?" If you become more fatigued with exercise, then your fatigue is probably associated with a deficiency syndrome. If, however, you always feel better with exercise, then your fatigue is the result of a stagnation syndrome. The possible individualized diagnoses include the following:

Kidney Deficiency—In addition to fatigue, the symptoms associated with weak Kidneys include low-back pain, knee soreness, frequent urination, incontinence in severe cases, spermatorrhea, premature ejaculation, and leukorrhea. The signs include a pale tongue and a thready, weak pulse.

If Kidney Yang is weak, there may be feelings of cold in the lumbar area, cold limbs, impotence, infertility, and tinnitus.

If Kidney Yin is weak, we may find symptoms such as afternoon fevers, night sweats, malar flush, hot palms and soles, and insomnia. Kidney Yin Deficiency is also associated with certain forms of tuberculosis and menopausal symptoms.

When the Kidney Jing is weak, there may be a lack of ovulation or a decrease in sperm production. Dryness often occurs, especially in the skin.

Spleen Qi and Xue Deficiency—In addition to fatigue, the symptoms of Spleen deficiency may include lack of appetite, nausea, flatulence, weight loss, and decrease in muscle mass and strength. Fluid retention and swelling may occur in the abdomen and extremities; there may be episodes of diarrhea.

If Spleen weakness leads to Xue Deficiency, there may be anemia. Symptoms include dry skin, a decrease in the menstrual flow, and lusterless skin. Sometimes these symptoms are also associated with Heart Qi Deficiency, which can lead to shortness of breath, difficulty walking up stairs, irregular heartbeat, and palpitations.

Spleen Yang Deficiency—In addition to fatigue a person may have watery diarrhea, often with whole particles of food in the stool.

Liver Qi Stagnation—The Liver Organ System is responsible for regulating the smooth flow of Qi throughout the body. If fatigue is triggered by stress—emotional, environmental, chemical, or physical—the Liver may not be able to satisfactorily regulate Qi.

2. You will also want to visit a Western doctor for a blood test to determine whether you have an undiagnosed infection that is causing the fatigue—for example, MAC causes extreme fatigue. You should also discuss potential reactions to current medications and treatments that might be causing the response.

3. Once your practitioners have tried to determine the source of the fatigue you will want to coordinate your treatments so they work together to build your stamina.

Self-care Program for Fatigue

In addition to the guidelines in the Basic Comprehensive HIV+ Treatment Program:

Rest and Sleep

It may seem obvious: If you're tired, you should rest. But many people try to fight chronic fatigue by ignoring its ravages and end up wearing themselves down. As a result they don't have the resources they need to combat the exhaustion efficiently. True, it is important to fight against the depression associated with unremitting fatigue and to retain a determined attitude. However, while you keep a strong mental and spiritual outlook, you must accept the physical demands of exhaustion: Rest is essential. For those with Epstein-Barr or CFIDS, a leave of absence from work is often mandatory in order to allow the body to recover. This is smart medicine, not defeat.

Diet

Some elements of chronic fatigue may be associated with food allergies. Therefore, an elimination diet that removes common allergens is a good place to start. For two weeks do not eat dairy products, wheat, corn, citrus, and tomatoes. If fatigue is eliminated, after two weeks, reintroduce these items, one per week, into your diet. If the fatigue returns, then you know to permanently eliminate the food.

Exercise

Those with severe fatigue syndromes may not feel as though they can exercise, but Qi Gong breathing and Qi-stimulating movements can be done with minimal exertion and still produce substantial benefits.

Try a modified arm swing (page 111) while doing Buddha's Breath. As strength returns, you can increase your routine, always sticking with the breathing practices. The best way to gauge if you're ready for a more active workout is to ask yourself: Could I walk comfortably at a steady pace for 20 minutes? If the answer is yes, then a daily 20-minute Qi Gong workout can provide the Qi-nurturing stimulation you need. It is essential that you not be depleted by the activity, so be wary of pushing yourself too hard.

Self-moxibustion

For stagnant or deficient Qi, moxibustion is beneficial. Concentrate on Stomach 36, Spleen 6, Large Intestine 10, and Ren 4, 6, 12. Have a partner moxa Urinary Bladder 13 for the Lung, Urinary Bladder 20 for the Spleen, and Urinary Bladder 23 for the Kidney—they're spots you can't reach by yourself. (For locations of the points, see pages 96–102.)

Ear Massage Points

Take 10 minutes, once a day, to massage Ear Sympathetic, Ear Kidney, Ear Lung (see page 104).

- For fatigue with digestion problems—Ear Stomach and Ear Spleen.
- For fatigue related to negative side effects of medications—Ear Liver.

Self-massage

The Qi Gong torso and belly massages (pages 119–120) will help stimulate Qi and give you a calm, steady boost of energy.

Other self-massage acupoints to focus on include Stomach 36, Kidney 3, Large Intestine 4, and Lung 7 (see pages 96–102).

Practitioner-Assisted Care Program for Fatigue

Herbs

All herbal preparations should be taken only under the supervision of a trained practitioner or medical doctor, with the exception of those few items listed in the Medicine Cabinet in Appendix 3.

Each syndrome associated with fatigue calls for its own herbal prescription.

- *Kidney Yang Deficiency*—Ba Wei Di Huang Wan or Golden Book Tea; Rehmannia 8; gecko-based Gejie Nourishing Pills from Yulin Drug in Kwangsi, China.
- *Severe Kidney Yin Deficiency*—Zhi Bai Di Wang Wan, or Eight Flavor Tea; Rehmannia 9; Temper Fire.

The primary herb in all but the Gejie pills is Rehmannia, an herb known to replenish the Kidney Yin. *Warning:* These formulas may cause digestive problems in people with a weakened Spleen System.

- *Kidney Essence Deficiency*—Gejie Nourishing Pills; Astra Essence by Health Concerns; Placenta Compound Restorative Pills from Bai-Yuen-Shan in Guang Zhou, China.
- *Spleen Deficiency*—Enhance, Four Gentlemen Tea, Six Gentlemen Tea.

Four Gentlemen may be prescribed strictly for strengthening the body's energy. Six Gentlemen has additional herbs to strengthen digestion as well as increase energy. The main ingredients are astragalus and ginseng or codonopsis. Enhance includes the Six Gentlemen formula but is designed specifically to target immune deficiency associated with viral disease and fatigue.

If the Spleen Deficiency is associated with diarrhea: Central Qi Tea (Bu Zhong Yi Qi Tang), Arouse Vigor from K'an, Clearing and Qi from Health Concerns, Astragalus and Ginseng Formula from Zand.

• *Xue Deficiency*—Eight Precious Pills (also called Women's Precious Pills), Tang Kwei Gin, Marrow Plus (particularly for fatigue associated with AZT or other anemia-causing drugs, chemotherapy, or radiation).

• *Liver Qi Stagnation*—Bupleurum Sedative Pill (Xiao Yao Wan) from Guang Zhou, China, K'an Relaxed Wanderer from K'an, Woman's Balance from Health Concerns.

If the Liver Qi Stagnation triggers depression, take Bupleurum and Dragon Bone, or Ease Plus from Health Concerns. If the disharmony deepens into Liver invading Spleen with such symptoms as flatulence and digestive problems, use Shu Gan Wan formula.

Acupuncture and Moxibustion

Receive acupuncture and moxibustion one to three times a week for severe fatigue and associated symptoms; the treatment depends on the individual diagnosis, but in each case an intensive routine for three to four weeks is recommended. Thereafter, a regular schedule of monthly treatments can help maintain strength and vigor. Moxibustion will follow the individualized diagnosis that guides acupuncture.

PROGRAM SEVEN: KAPOSI'S SARCOMA

Once considered a form of cancer, Kaposi's sarcoma (KS) now appears to be a sexually transmitted viral disease. (In this country it has primarily been seen in gay men, while in Africa it is predominately transmitted heterosexually.) In the 1980s, approximately 35 percent of all people with AIDS had been diagnosed with KS; the incidence of the disease has dropped dramatically to 14 percent in recent years. The symptoms of KS include purple lesions on the skin and internal organs and mucous membranes caused by the proliferation of the cells in the walls of the blood vessels and spindle cells from smooth muscles. When the lesions are internal they can occur in the gastrointestinal tract, lungs, spleen, heart, and lymph nodes. In addition, KS produces fatigue, lack of appetite, and difficulty with digestion. Other symptoms are associated with the organ system that is involved. There is no known preventive treatment, and current Western therapy includes chemotherapy or interferon therapy for internal lesions, and for skin lesions, cryotherapy (freezing of the lesion to remove it), chemotherapy, surgical removal, and sometimes radiation.

Treatment Options for Kaposi's Sarcoma

1. Obtain a Chinese medicine diagnosis. The syndromes involved include stagnant Xue (blood) and, when associated with swelling in the legs, Kidney Qi or Spleen Qi Deficiency.

2. Obtain a Western medical diagnosis; to determine internal organ involvement a biopsy may be necessary. To avoid damage from proliferative tissue impinging on organ function, prompt treatment is advised.

3. The combination of Western and Chinese medicine offers a strong therapeutic base: Chinese medicine can help ameliorate the side effects of chemotherapy and help ease dermatological problems associated with skin lesions.

Self-care Program for Kaposi's Sarcoma

In addition to the guidelines in the Basic Comprehensive HIV+ Treatment Program:

Moxibustion

Self-moxibustion on Xue Stagnation points, particularly Spleen 10 and Large Intestine 11, plus over any lesions that are not open or oozing (see pages 96–102).

Massage

Although massage may be uncomfortable, it is advisable because it helps decrease pain and ease swelling in legs and feet. Use a massage oil made of 1 cup almond oil to ¹/₂ teaspoon evening primrose oil. For cold arms and legs, use cinnamon oil. These rubs are particularly useful as skin thickens and hardens as a result of the disease or from chemotherapy.

Practitioner-Assisted Care Program
for Kaposi's Sarcoma

Your practitioner will design a treatment program based on the symptoms you experience in relation to the disease, whether they are respiratory, gastrointestinal, or dermatological. The treatment may evolve during the course of the disease. For help in managing the repercussions of chemotherapy, use Marrow Plus to strengthen bone marrow and Sai Mei An and Tien Chi Powder, both available at Chinese herb stores, as topical salves for irritated areas. To make a salve from one of these herbs combine it with an equal portion of evening primrose oil. (Do not use this mixture for a general, whole-body massage oil.)

PROGRAM EIGHT: SINUSITIS

Sinusitis, the chronic irritation and infection of the sinuses, is one of the most persistent problems associated with HIV. It may arise as a result of a bacterial, viral, or fungal infection in the sinuses; as a symptom associated with PCP, MAC, and other HIV-related infections; or from chronic allergies. The result can be persistent head pain, sore throat, lowering of overall stamina, cough, lung congestion, ear infections, and hearing problems and fatigue. Treatment is tailored to the specific causes, but there are some general Chinese medicine treatments that are effective in controlling symptoms. Western medicine offers antibiotics and antihistamines and decongestants but can do little to knock out chronic HIV-related sinus problems.

Treatment Options for Sinusitis

1. Obtain a Chinese medicine diagnosis and begin sinus wash and steaming immediately (page 167).

2. Consult with your Western physician to determine whether the sinus condition is related to an acute infection that demands immediate antibiotic or other treatment.

3. Always keep practitioners informed about your at-home self-care practices and the treatment you are receiving from each of them.

Self-care Program for Sinusitis
In addition to the guidelines in the Basic Comprehensive HIV+ Treatment Program:

Diet
To determine if food allergies are triggering your sinus symptoms, a basic elimination diet will help identify the possible irritants. For two to three weeks eliminate dairy products, sugar, caffeine, alcohol, tomatoes, eggs, citrus, and wheat from your diet. Then add them back in, one per week. If you find your sinus-related symptoms increase, you may be wise to eliminate the offending food from your diet altogether for at least several months. Eventually, you may be able to reintroduce it into your diet in small quantities.

Self-acupressure
To relieve pain, press gently but firmly on the inner corner of the eyebrow beside the nose; below the center of the eye in the hollow of the cheekbone; outside the outer corner of the eye; and on the hand on Large Intestine 4, which is located on the webbing between the thumb and the index finger. While you give yourself a facial treatment, you may want to place a drop of

White Flower Oil on the tip of your nose to help open nasal passages. (Be very careful not to get any near or in your eyes.)

Hand and foot reflexology and ear massage on areas associated with head, forehead, and sinuses are also beneficial (see pages 104, 122–123).

Sinus Wash

This simple, inexpensive home remedy can have a profound healing effect on chronic sinus infections, allergy-related congestion and irritation, chronic cough, and postnasal drip if done consistently for two to three months.

1. Make a salt solution for use in a glass sinus irrigator or rubber sinus bulb (available at most pharmacies). Use nonchlorinated, filtered, or boiled water and kosher or sea salt: $1/2$ to 1 teaspoon per cup of water. Work up to 2 teaspoons salt per cup. Note: If even the mild solution of saltwater is too irritating, irrigate sinuses with pure filtered water.

2. Breathe in three to four drops per nostril, tilting head back and holding opposite nostril closed. Repeat three to five times on each side. Be careful not to force the solution up into the sinuses with too much pressure. The areas of damaged tissue will feel a sharp sensation for a few seconds. Over time the sensation will fade as the tissue begins to heal. The sinuses will begin to drain as the old buildup loosens. There may be slight amount of blood in the discharge. (If you have an ear infection, do not use the sinus wash until it is cleared up.)

Facial Steam

To steam with herbs: Infuse a basin of boiling water with one to three drops of White Flower Oil, red thyme oil (particularly good for bacterial infections), and/or eucalyptus oil. Lean over steaming basin and cover your head with a towel to capture the steam. Be careful not to burn skin or tender nasal passages. Keep your eyes closed to avoid stinging sensation. Steam for three to four minutes. Electric steam inhalers are also available at local pharmacies.

Practitioner-Assisted Care for Sinusitis

Herbs

All herbal preparations should be taken only under the supervision of a trained practitioner or medical doctor, with the exception of those few items listed in the Medicine Cabinet in Appendix 3.

Using herbs to steam and irrigate the sinuses is highly effective.

- Sinus irrigation—Pi Yen Chin is an herbal liquid that your practitioner may prescribe as a wash for nasal passages and sinuses.
- Sinus tea and steam—Many times a practitioner will create an individualized acute sinusitis tea in a cooked formula. You can both drink this

and use it to steam your sinuses. Here's an example of one that is used to remove damp/stop cough/open sinuses: Xing Ren (apricot seed), Pi Pa Ye (eriobotryae), Jie Geng (platycodon), Zi Wan (asteris root), Chen Pi (citrus peel), Lu Gen (phragmites), Ma Huang (ephedra), Gan Cao (licorice root), Xin Yi Hua (magnolia flower), Cang Er Zi (xanthium fruit), Bai Ji Li or Ci Ji Li (tribulous fruit).

Herbal pill formulas for sinusitis include:

- For runny nose and allergies—Minor Blue Dragon Pills.
- For damp blocking sinuses—Clear Air.
- For sinus obstruction—Pe Min Kan Wan (Use Plum Flower brand only. Others contain unregulated pharmaceuticals).

Acupuncture

- For blocked ears—Triple Burner 17 or 21 and Gallbladder 2; Small Intestine 19.
- For digestive problems related to postnasal drip—Ren 12.
- For common cold symptoms—Large Intestine 4; Lung 7; Triple Burner 5; Gallbladder 20. In addition, put a small amount of White Flower Oil under the nose during treatment.
- To ease sinus pain and open sinuses—Large Intestine 4, 20; Stomach 1, 2, 3, 44; Du 22, 23; Urinary Bladder 2; Gallbladder 20.

PROGRAM NINE: SKIN CONDITIONS

HIV/AIDS and associated syndromes create a wide variety of dermatological conditions, from allergic rashes to psoriasis, nerve-related itching—called pruritis—to skin lesions. Some of the skin problems are symptoms of underlying disorders, others are unexplained responses to HIV infection, and others are reactions to medications.

Seborrheic dermatitis is characterized by scaly skin patches, lesions around the nose and eyebrows and behind the ears. This non-infectious condition appears to be related to falling CD4+ cell counts. Treatment is difficult but ketoconazole applied as a cream or taken orally is successful in about 25 percent of patients.

Psoriasis is at least twice as prevalent among people who are HIV-positive as among the general population, leading to speculation that it is related to immune function. Lesions are often in the groin and on the scalp, hands, and feet. Western medical treatment uses corticosteroids, cyclosporin, and ultraviolet light.

Other HIV-related skin conditions include *folliculitis,* in which the hair follicles become infected and/or severely itchy; *photosensitivity,* in response to drug therapy and to HIV infection; *porphyria cutanea tarda,* which is hyperpigmentation of skin and the formation of small white blisters when exposed to sun; and *xeroderma,* dry skin with scaly patches and a rash that comes and goes.

Chinese diagnosis is completely individualized and a large number of variations may be diagnosed. The main ones are the following:

Dryness, which is easily irritated, dry skin without redness and flaking.

Heat in Xue (blood) is associated with pruritis, red, itchy rashes, inflamed patches, and areas with stagnant Xue such as appear in association with Kaposi's sarcoma. It is sometimes accompanied by fever.

Liver Heat/Damp Heat is associated with red, itching, oozing rashes or patches. It may be accompanied by nausea, fatigue, and pain on the sides of the torso.

Treatment Options for Skin Conditions

1. Obtain a Chinese medicine diagnosis. Since there are so many possible underlying causes, a careful evaluation must be made.

2. Consult your Western practitioner to see if a drug reaction is involved and discuss your options and repercussions. Explore the possibility that the skin condition is related to an undiagnosed opportunistic infection and determine whether drug therapy is required immediately to prevent further complications.

3. Always keep practitioners informed about your at-home self-care practices and the treatment you are receiving from each of them.

Self-care Program for Skin Conditions

In addition to the guidelines in the Basic Comprehensive HIV+ Treatment Program:

Herb Washes for Sebhorrheic Dermatitis, Dry Skin (Xeroderma), and Psoriasis

For the scalp—Combine 1 quart of chamomile tea and ¼ cup flaxseed oil, evening primrose oil, and/or tea tree oil. Mix medium-warm tea and oil in basin and plunge scalp into liquid for as long as it remains warm. Rinse with filtered warm water. Wrap head in towel and leave for 30 minutes. Rinse with hot chamomile tea and air-dry.

For the rest of the skin—Create a warm bath infused with chamomile. Place a cup of chamomile flowers on a square of cheesecloth and tie up ends securely. Allow bath to fill over the cup. Add ¼ cup oil—be careful getting in and out of tub; the oil makes it very slippery. Soak for 20 minutes. Pat dry gently; don't rub all the oil off.

Herbal Body Rubs

- For dry skin and Kaposi's lesions—Rub a solution of 10 to 15 drops of evening primrose oil mixed in ¼ cup virgin olive oil over affected areas. Leave on skin for at least 45 minutes. Pat dry with soft gauze squares. For very irritated or dry areas, place gauze patch over oil-covered area like a bandage and secure with tape or clear plastic wrap. Leave overnight.
- For rashes, itchy skin, and sun-related reactions—Use an Aveeno oatmeal soak (see page 117).
- Tea tree oil and calendula salve, a homeopathic remedy, are also useful on raw areas.

Diet

In addition to the basic natural foods diet—low in fats, sugars, and red meats, high in whole grains and vegetables—make sure you drink at least 32 ounces (four cups) of water a day initially. After ten days increase it to 48 ounces (six cups).

- *For Excess Heat syndromes*—Avoid garlic, turkey, and heavy oils.
- *For Excess Dampness syndromes*—Avoid dairy products, fried foods, and alcohol and coffee.

Exercise

Qi Gong (see page 109) is particularly important because of its effect on the Lung and Liver Organ Systems.

Practitioner-Assisted Program for Skin Conditions

Herbal Formulas

All herbal preparations should be taken only under the supervision of a trained practitioner or medical doctor, with the exception of those few items listed in the Medicine Cabinet in Appendix 3.

For general skin rashes and allergic reactions, the following herbal formulas are used: Armadillo Pills; Forsythia 18; Spring Wind Ointment; Zaocys Tablets; Yin Chiao Chieh Tu Pien. An example of a raw herb combo is Lian Qiao, Da Qing Ye, Ban Lan Gen, Tu Fu Ling, Fu Ling, Huang Qi, Tian Hua Fen.

- For photosensitivity and reactions to sunlight—Take the herb formula called Coptis Purge Fire (see Appendix 3) to clear heat and dampness.

- For drug reactions—If possible, stop taking the drug. If this is not possible, use Armadillo Pills, which can be obtained in Chinese herb stores.
- For sinusitis-related skin conditions—Use the herbal formula Xanthium Relieve Surface to ease rashes and raw skin around nose.

Acupuncture

- General treatment for healthy skin—Lung 7, Large Intestine 11, Stomach 36, Urinary Bladder 13 and 20, and Gallbladder 20. With a heat condition, also Liver 2.
- Ear acupuncture—Shenmen, Sympathetic; Liver and Lung (see diagram, page 104).

Supplements

- Organic borage and flax oil—1 to 2 tablespoons a day.
- Powdered vitamin E—800 to 1,200 IU a day.
- Zinc picolinate—There is some debate over the use of zinc by people who are HIV-positive. For more information consult publications and books by Mary Romeyn, M.D., and Lark Lands, Ph.D., a nutritional consultant specializing in HIV-related problems (see Appendix 5).

Massage
If there are no open lesions, rub irritated area with cooling oils such as White Flower Oil. Other effective emollients include sesame oil for dry skin and Aubrey Organics Evening Primrose Complexion and Body Lotion.

PROGRAM TEN: CHRONIC DIARRHEA AND ASSOCIATED GASTROINTESTINAL PROBLEMS

Severe chronic diarrhea affects 30 to 50 percent of everyone who is HIV-positive, and the results are profoundly serious. Not only does it produce extreme discomfort, making it difficult at times to have a normal social life, but it can destroy your appetite, deprive you of needed nutritional support, and cause severe weight loss and wasting. Furthermore, chronic diarrhea irritates the intestinal tract, making it even more susceptible to additional problems, and lowers overall strength and weakens the immune system. That's why you must act immediately to stop diarrhea before it becomes chronic and to hold chronic diarrhea in check even as you continue to search for an explanation of its cause.

Finding out the trigger can be extremely difficult. Diarrhea can occur for many reasons:

- HIV—The virus itself is thought to stimulate diarrhea at various stages.
- Protozoal infections—Cryptosporidium triggers the most severe diarrhea.
- Parasites—Giardia is a major and frequently overlooked cause.
- Viral infections—CMV (cytomegalovirus), for example, does frequently lodge in the gastrointestinal tract.
- Other opportunistic infections—MAC *(Mycobacterium avium* complex) is often associated with diarrhea.
- Candida overgrowth—Antibiotic therapy or a weakened immune system may allow candida to flourish. This fungal infection may block digestion and mask simultaneous infection with parasites.
- Stress and depression—We all have experienced a nervous stomach when some stressful event is looming before us. For people who are HIV-positive, stress and related depression is often a constant companion: Worries about having the disease can overwhelm even the strongest determination to remain optimistic and in control.
- Food poisoning (bacterial infections)—Salmonella, campylobacter, and listeria bacteria are the most common varieties and people with HIV are far more susceptible to them and develop severe, acute diarrhea as a result. It is estimated that HIV-positive people are 200 to 300 times more likely to develop listeria infection and 20 times more likely to contract salmonella or campylobacter. In addition, salmonella also triggers recurrent episodes once initial antibiotic treatment is completed.
- Other possible causes—Lactose intolerance, excessive fat consumption, food allergies, excess coffee intake, nicotine or other "recreational drugs," medications for HIV-related syndromes, and antiviral medications.

In addition, because people with HIV are susceptible to the various causes of diarrhea, a chronic case may be the result of not one but several parasites or of candidiasis combined with parasites, or food allergies, a drug reaction, and a viral infection. Consequently, effective treatment must address each factor involved. And the therapy must not itself cause diarrhea.

Treatment Options for Diarrhea

1. Obtain a Chinese medicine diagnosis to determine the underlying cause of the diarrhea. Possible diagnoses for chronic diarrhea include:

- Spleen Qi and Yang Deficiency—Often associated with parasite infection, these syndromes are characterized by diarrhea with watery stools with undigested food, a feeling of being chilled or cold, a lack of appetite, and a swollen, pale tongue and slow or tight pulse.
- Dampness invading the Spleen—Characterized by flatulence, loose stool, swollen limbs and abdomen, swollen tongue, and a thready pulse.

- Damp Heat in Spleen—Characterized by loose, strong-smelling stools, fever, nausea, swollen abdomen, slippery fast pulse, red swollen tongue.
- Large Intestine Damp Heat—Characterized by loose stools or alternating loose stools and constipation, cramping in lower abdomen, mucus and or blood in stool, fever, red tongue, slippery, rapid pulse.
- Liver/Gallbladder Damp Heat—Characterized by loose stools, pain along the sides of the torso, fever—perhaps alternating with chills—a bitter taste in the mouth, nausea, headache, purplish red tongue, wiry or slippery pulse.

2. Obtain a Western medical diagnosis. Have a stool culture done at a top-notch lab such as Great Smokies (see Appendix 8). Many places miss hard-to-find parasites or other microorganisms that are responsible for the diarrhea. And don't forget there may be several simultaneous causes of your chronic diarrhea: Get tested for allergies; eliminate caffeine, dairy, and recreational drugs; cut fat intake to 25 percent of daily calories, raise protein to 20 percent, and raise grains and legumes to 55 percent. Have your doctor evaluate the possibility that your medications are contributing to or even causing your condition. Discuss options.

3. Always keep practitioners informed about your self-care practices and the treatment you are receiving from each of them.

Self-care Program for Diarrhea

In addition to the guidelines in the Basic Comprehensive HIV+ Treatment Program:

Diet

To help ease diarrhea, whatever the cause, avoid all cold or raw foods, spicy food, coffee, chocolate, and all dark soft drinks. Add to your diet a daily serving of white rice (not brown); barley to reduce dampness; green and black tea as astringents to help reduce water content of stools.

Exercise

Do 30 minutes of Qi Gong, including breathing exercise, as frequently as possible. Regular aerobic exercise, such as speed-walking, jogging, swimming, or a step aerobics class, helps promote healthy digestion as well.

Meditation

To reduce the contribution that stress may be making to your gastrointestinal troubles and to help strengthen and regulate Qi, do the long meditation on page 112 at least three times a week—every day is best.

Self-massage

An abdominal massage helps harmonize the Large and Small Intestine, Liver, Spleen, Stomach, and Gallbladder. To increase the massage's effectiveness, use a cinnamon-infused massage oil and follow the steps for the belly massage on page 120.

Moxibustion

Do salt-moxibustion in the navel once a day. Other points that are important include Stomach 25, 36, 37; Spleen 9, 6; Ren 6 (see pages 96–102).

Practitioner-Assisted Program for Diarrhea

Herbs

All herbal preparations should be taken only under the supervision of a trained practitioner or medical doctor—with the exception of those few items listed in the Medicine Cabinet in Appendix 3.

- For Spleen Qi and Yang Deficiency—Source Qi, Bu Zhong Yi Qi Wan, Shen Ling Bai Zhu Wan.
- With parasites—Artestatin, always at a reduced dose and in conjunction with Enhance or Source Qi.
- For Damp Cold associated with Cryptosporidiosis—Garlic pills, three to six a day with food; Source Qi.
- For Dampness associated with antibiotic therapy—Phellostatin.
- Herbal enemas for Cryptosporidiosis—Practitioner-designed only.

Acupuncture

Recommended one to three times a week during acute or severe phase; once a week thereafter. The points that are most effective in stopping chronic and acute diarrhea include Large Intestine 4, 10; Spleen 6, 9; Stomach 25, 36, 37.

Moxibustion

Moxibustion is always used with deficiency-related diarrhea. The points to concentrate on are Ren 8 (navel); Stomach 25, 36; Spleen 6, 9 (see pages 96–102).

Supplements

In addition to the regular program, add a daily dose of psyllium, which is in products such as Fiber-All. Do not use whole seeds.

PROGRAM ELEVEN: HEPATITIS

Hepatitis, inflammation of the liver, can occur as a result of a viral infection or as a reaction to medication or chronic abuse of alcohol. It may also be related to the opportunistic infection cytomegalovirus. There are several varieties: hepatitis A, B, C, D, and E. Hepatitis A is generally contracted through ingestion of fecal matter in contaminated food or water and does not hang on and become a chronic disease. There is now a vaccine available.

Hepatitis B is transmitted sexually and through exchange of blood, particularly needle sharing. Contracting hepatitis B while HIV-positive appears to hasten the progression to AIDS. Furthermore, the presence of HIV appears to make it vastly more difficult to treat the hepatitis virus, and the disease often progresses to chronic liver disease, causing cirrhosis and liver cancer. A vaccine for hepatitis B is available, and those who are HIV-positive and hepatitis antibody–negative should strongly consider taking advantage of this protection. Hepatitis C and the other strains appear to be spread through contaminated needles, transfusions, and possibly sexual contact. Treatment for B and C is alpha interferon, but it is not effective for the vast majority of those treated.

Chinese medicine views liver inflammation as one of six possible syndromes:

• Damp Heat Liver/Gallbladder—Characterized by discomfort in the top of the shoulders and rib cage, a bitter taste in the mouth, poor appetite, scanty dark urine, jaundice, fever and chills, and emotional lability. When the Gallbladder System is also involved, there are additional symptoms, including Shen disturbances leading to anger and impulsiveness, uncertainty and hesitation, and lack of strong character. In acute viral hepatitis the tongue is characterized as red and swollen with yellow fur, and there is a wiry or slippery pulse.

• Liver Qi Stagnation—Characterized by uncomfortable feelings in the chest and between the ribs, abdominal distention, restlessness, depression, and a quick temper. The tongue is normal or purplish; the pulse is slippery.

• Damp Heat Spleen—Characterized by loss of appetite; fullness in the stomach; scanty, dark urine and tiredness; occasionally a thirst without the desire to drink; itchy skin and fever. The tongue is characterized as swollen and reddish with a yellow greasy fur and the pulse is slippery and fast. Damp Heat Spleen is usually associated with acute viral hepatitis.

• Damp Cold Spleen—Characterized by lack of appetite, watery stools, a lusterless, yellow face, fatigue, and no thirst. The tongue is swollen and pale and the pulse is tight and slippery.

• Qi and Xue Deficiency—Liver Qi Deficiency causing Qi Deficiency throughout the body is characterized by a failure in the joints, malaise, shallow breathing, a lack of forcefulness in voice, and spontaneous sweating. When combined with Xue Deficiency the symptoms include dry skin, shrunken liver, a pale tongue, and a deep, weak, thready pulse.

• Xue Stagnation—Stagnant Liver Xue is characterized by fixed, sharp, stabbing pains and palpable masses. Women's symptoms also include missed periods, menstrual clotting, and cramps.

Treatment Options for Hepatitis

1. Obtain a Chinese medicine diagnosis and begin treatment promptly to protect liver from further damage. Lab tests should be taken to test for liver enzyme levels and chronic hepatitis B and C. If there are acute symptoms test for hepatitis A as well.

2. Obtain a Western diagnosis to determine the viral strain. You also want to track the impact of the hepatitis infection on your overall health and on your immune system by having regular blood tests and other monitoring evaluations. Discuss the pros and cons of Western drug therapy with your doctor and work together to determine the best treatment for your individual case.

3. Always keep practitioners informed of your self-care practices and of the treatment you are receiving from each of them.

Self-care Program for Hepatitis

In addition to the guidelines in the Basic Comprehensive HIV+ Treatment Program:

Diet

With heat syndromes, avoid eating hot or warm foods such as ginger, soybean oil, trout. Also avoid foods that are warm, including anchovies, basil, bay leaf, black pepper, brown sugar, butter, capers, cherries, chestnuts, chicken, garlic, fresh ginger, mussels, mutton, onions, peaches, pine nuts, rosemary, shrimp, strawberries, sweet potatoes, vinegar, and walnuts.

Eliminate alcohol and coffee from your diet, and with excess dampness, avoid fried foods and dairy products.

Massage

An abdominal massage helps harmonize the Large and Small Intestine, Liver, Spleen, Stomach, and Gallbladder. To increase the massage's effectiveness, use a cinnamon-infused massage oil.

Practitioner-Assisted Program for Hepatitis

Herbs

All herbal preparations should be taken only under the supervision of a trained practitioner or medical doctor, with the exception of those few items listed in the Medicine Cabinet in Appendix 3.

As a general herbal therapy for chronic hepatitis, in addition to Enhance or Tremella American Ginseng and Clear Heat, you may take:

- Ecliptex two to three times a day.
- Silymarin 80 percent concentrate—One to four pills a day.
- Li Gan Pian—For use with high liver enzymes.

For other conditions associated with hepatitis, try the following:

- For Damp Heat Liver—Long Dan Xie Gan Wan, Coptis Purge Fire.
- For Damp Heat Gallbladder—Li Dan Pian.
- For Damp Cold Spleen—Shen Ling Bai Zhu Wan.
- For Liver Qi Stagnation—Woman's Balance, Xiao Yao Wan, Shu Gan Wan.
- For Qi and Xue Deficiency—Eight Precious Pills, Wu Ji Bai Feng Wan (Black Chicken Pills).
- For Xue Stagnation—Yan Hu Suo Wan, Channel Flow.

Acupuncture

Points for chronic hepatitis are Liver 3; Large Intestine 4; Urinary Bladder 18, 19, 20; Gallbladder 24 and Liver 14; and Stomach 36 (with deficiency). In addition, there are special Korean acupuncture points used for chronic hepatitis that are located at the level of the thoracic vertebrae 10, 11, and 12, halfway between the Du and Urinary Bladder channels.

- For Damp Heat Liver—Gallbladder 34, Liver 3, Ren 12, Spleen 6, Ear Liver, Ear Gallbladder, Yin Tang.
- For Damp Heat Spleen—Spleen 6, 9; Ren 12; Yin Tang.
- For Damp Cold Spleen—See Moxibustion, page 178.
- For Liver Qi Stagnation—Large Intestine 3; Gallbladder 34.
- For Qi and Xue Deficiency—Stomach 36; Spleen 6; Urinary Bladder 20, 21, 23.
- For Xue Stagnation—Spleen 10, Large Intestine 11.

Moxibustion

- For Damp Cold Spleen and Qi and Xue Deficiency—Stomach 36 and Spleen 6; with nausea, add Ren 12. (See pages 96–102 for location of points.)

Supplements

Maintain a beta-carotene dosage of 5,000 to 10,000 IU a day.

PROGRAM TWELVE: FEVERS AND NIGHT SWEATS

Fevers and night sweats are associated with primary HIV infection and appear as a result of the many opportunistic infections and disorders that are related to lowered immune function. Fever is evidence of the body's fight against disease, but it can do great harm: depleting strength, dehydrating the body, and, when chronic, disturbing sleep patterns, causing psychological distress and loss of appetite. If you have a fever over 101 degrees Fahrenheit for more than two days, you may want to consult your Western physician to make sure you are not in an acute phase of an opportunistic infection that requires immediate treatment.

Treatment Options for Fever and Night Sweats

1. Obtain a Chinese medicine diagnosis of the fevers. Fevers, particularly those related to the primary HIV infection, may be a sign of:

Excessive Liver Fire—This is often a result of worsening stagnant Liver Qi and is associated with eye pain; red eyes; sharp pain in the chest; scanty, yellow urine; quick temper; dry stools; and eventually, if it moves on to interior Liver Wind, fever with convulsions and loss of consciousness.

Deficient Liver Yin—Chronic low-grade fevers, night sweats, dizziness, headaches, and numb limbs, as well as a quick temper and dry mouth and throat, are symptoms of this disharmony.

Heat invading the Xue—This is characterized by severe rashes and bloody stools or urine. High fever can lead to coma.

If heat invading Xue is due to a Xue Deficiency, then symptoms may include dry skin, fatigue, a pale face and pale tongue with red edges, and a weak, fast pulse.

2. Obtain a Western diagnosis. Tests for MAC and PCP are usually recommended. Other screening tests may reveal additional bacterial or viral infections. Also, discuss with your doctor the possibility that drug reactions may be fueling the fevers. If the fever is associated with the primary HIV infection, treatment may center on lowering the fever with aspirin and cool compresses. There isn't much else that can be done.

3. Always keep practitioners informed about your self-care practices and the treatment you are receiving from each practitioner.

Self-care Program for Fevers and Night Sweats

In addition to the guidelines in the Basic Comprehensive HIV + Treatment Program:

Diet

To help quell Internal Heat, avoid foods that are categorized as hot, including ginger, soybean oil, and trout. Avoid also foods that are warm, including anchovies, basil, bay leaf, black pepper, brown sugar, butter, capers, cherries, chestnuts, chicken, garlic, fresh ginger, mussels, mutton, onions, peaches, pine nuts, rosemary, shrimp, strawberries, sweet potatoes, vinegar, and walnuts.

Add more cool and cold foods to your diet, including apples, bananas, barley, buckwheat, celery, cucumber, eggplant, gluten, lettuce, millet, mushrooms, pears, peppermint, sesame oil, soybeans, spinach, Swiss chard, tangerines, tofu, watercress, wheat, asparagus, clams, kelp, mangoes, tomatoes, watermelons.

Other beneficial foods include wheat congee (page 69); Swiss chard juice; Chinese white cucumber tea made from pureed and strained white cucumber with 1/2 teaspoon of sugar; clam broth with clams.

Meditation

Peaceful meditation can provide tranquillity and allow the body to dissipate heat. Follow the routine on page 112.

Soaks

Lukewarm and tepid soaks (never cold) can help lower body temperature. If you become chilled you will only increase the fever, so make sure that you are comfortable at all times.

Recommended soaks include the peppermint tea and chamomile soaks on page 117. Another soothing soak is the lemon soak: Tie four lemons, quartered and squeezed gently to release the juice, into a cheesecloth "tea bag." Steep in bathtub for 20 minutes.

Practitioner-Assisted Program for Fevers and Night Sweats

Herbs
All herbal preparations should be taken only under the supervision of a trained practitioner or medical doctor, with the exception of those few items listed in the Medicine Cabinet in Appendix 3.

For chronic, low-grade fevers of unknown origin or from primary HIV infection your practitioner may recommend the following:

- Tremella America Ginseng may be used for night sweats and afternoon fevers and Yin Deficiency syndromes.
- Clear Heat may be used for sweating with fever.
- Da Bu Yin Wan may be used for Yin Deficient afternoon fevers or night sweats.
- Ginseng tea may be used to help restore Yang in the Lower Triple Burner and end sweating.

Acupuncture
For Yin Deficiency fevers with sweating add specific diagnosis related to the fever, Heart 6, and Kidney 7.

PROGRAM THIRTEEN: ADDICTION AND HIV/AIDS

Transmission of HIV as a result of drug addiction and related behaviors is a rapidly growing problem that affects people of all ages, races, and ethnic groups and from every economic and social class. There are many innovative programs around the country that make a enormous effort to reach those who lives are in double jeopardy because of drug use and abuse. The program outlined in this section was developed by Carla Wilson, L.Ac., an addiction specialist, director of Quan Yin Healing Arts Center, and founder of Clinica el Rio de la Vida, a full-service Chinese medicine clinic serving HIV-infected people in the South Bronx, including those addicted to drugs.

Treatment Options for Drug and Alcohol Withdrawal
Addiction to and withdrawal from drugs has a great impact on the immune system and the mind/body/spirit of people with HIV/AIDS. To meet the challenge of treating this twofold health problem, Western medicine has joined with Chinese medicine in programs across the country to offer acupuncture that helps with the withdrawal and treatment process. This is one area in which even the most conventional medical practitioners have accepted the usefulness of Chinese medicine. Follow these steps:

1. Visit a Chinese medicine doctor and discuss your options for going through withdrawal using acupuncture and herbs to support you in the process. At the same time allow the practitioner to evaluate your HIV infection to determine the overall health of your mind/body/spirit and to identify any HIV-related infections or syndromes that might also be present.

Each form of addiction has a unique effect on the mind/body/spirit:

- Heroin (or heroin with alcohol and tobacco) is associated with Yin Damp disharmony.
- Psychedelic-drug abuse is associated with Yang Deficiency.
- Crack creates depletion of Yin and Lung Deficiency; after continuous use, Kidney depletion and adrenal exhaustion set in and the person may develop Kidney Qi Deficiency.
- Methamphetamine use is related to Yin Deficiency with dryness. In addition, crack and meth force Qi out from the central core of the body, unmooring the mind/body/spirit. Eventually this produces psychosis.
- Alcohol use leads to Dampness with Yin Deficiency and Liver Heat and/ or Qi Stagnation.

Initially the Spleen and Stomach are not involved in addictive syndromes, but because people who are using drugs often don't eat or take care of themselves well, nutritional levels plummet and digestion becomes impaired by the drug itself and through neglect.

When HIV infection is added to the health challenges caused by addiction, the Spleen and Stomach Systems (which are immediately affected by the HIV) are thrown into deeper disharmony than they would be otherwise. This leads to the development of multiple problems: vulnerability to tuberculosis, influenza, and even the common cold increases dramatically.

2. Visit a Western medical doctor; or a drug treatment clinic that offers acupuncture along with therapy and medical support.

3. Always keep practitioners informed about your at-home self-care practices and the treatment you are receiving from each practitioner.

Practitioner-Assisted Program for Drug and Alcohol Withdrawal

When someone comes into the clinic and asks for treatment for drug addiction, they are urged to follow the guidelines in the Basic Comprehensive HIV+ Treatment Program and to take two additional steps immediately:

1. Join a 12-step group or some other support group, plus obtain professional psychotherapy.

2. Receive acupuncture treatments every day for 10 to 30 days during withdrawal. Acupuncture must be used in combination with support and therapy programs. Moxibustion is not used because with addiction the body is already too hot. All supportive treatments must cool and calm. Then, if the person receiving treatment also suffers from chronic diarrhea or neuropathy, moxibustion may be added to the treatment plan at a later time.

Acupuncture

Ear acupuncture, first pioneered for addictive therapy at Lincoln Detox Center in the Bronx, is now widely used in programs across the country. The main ear points include Ear Shenmen, Ear Sympathetic, Ear Liver, Ear Kidney, and Ear Lung. Acupuncture on the body focuses on Liver 3, Stomach 36, Yin Tang, and Du 20.

Herbs

All herbal preparations should be taken only under the supervision of a trained practitioner or medical doctor—with the exception of those few items listed in the Medicine Cabinet in Appendix 3.

During the withdrawal period herbs are used to promote sleep—so essential to a healthy recovery. Teas brewed from colt's foot and chamomile are recommended to be taken nightly. Herb formulas such as Ease Plus and Schizandra Dreams are sedatives that reduce withdrawal anxiety and ease insomnia.

Supplements

Follow the Basic Comprehensive HIV+ Treatment Program supplement recommendations daily, but pay special attention to improving eating habits so the bulk of your nutrition is from foods. Also, have a daily dose of some form of a fresh natural green juice made from wheat grass, parsley, celery, and/or spirulina (an easily assimilated protein that comes in a powder firm and is mixed into room-temperature water).

B vitamins are important during initial withdrawal, especially for alcohol detox.

Coenzyme Q_{10} and vitamin C to bowel tolerance help bolster overall immune strength. Ask your doctor or practitioner about taking selenium and other minerals.

Massage

Massage helps clear the lymph system and tissues of toxins and fluids. But not everyone can tolerate it during detoxification—some kinds of touch may be too intense or even painful. However, as soon as it is comfortable, an abdominal massage (see page 120) once a week helps heal Organ System damage and keeps Qi flowing through the channels.

Shiatsu/acupressure can help people who harbor anxiety in neck and shoulders. *Swedish* massage helps cleanse tissues and promotes relaxation. *Reiki* is a good alternative for those who do not want much touch. It can help move Qi and rebalance the body; often it helps people regain faith that good things are going on within their own bodies—so vital in the process of reclaiming yourself postaddiction. *Reflexology/foot massage* opens up Organ Systems and promotes circulation.

Self-Care Program for Drug and Alcohol Withdrawal

In addition to the guidelines in the Basic Comprehensive HIV + Treatment Program:

No one—or almost no one—can go through the overwhelming rigors of withdrawal from drugs or alcohol alone, especially while they are also contending with HIV infection. And even if they could, it's not a great idea. You want people to watch out for any physical complications that might affect the course of your HIV infection and to help prevent complications if possible. That said, there are some self-care techniques that you can use to help your transition off drugs.

Ear Self-Massage

The general detoxification points are Shenmen, Sympathetic, and Lung, plus Stomach on the left ear and Liver on the right ear (see the diagram on page 104). In addition:

- For alcohol detox—Ear Spleen and Ear Liver points. Add right Ear Lower Lung and left Ear Upper Lung.
- For crack detox—Add Du 20 (page 101).
- For tobacco smoking—Stick with Ear Shenmen and Ear Lung points.

Diet

Digestive upset from the addiction, from the withdrawal, and from the HIV infection itself can make dietary management a crucial part of the healing process.

- Create menus that contain easily assimilated protein foods such as chicken, fish, and cooked vegetables.
- Avoid all greasy and raw foods.
- Resist the urge to eat lots of sweets—with HIV infection that only encourages the overgrowth of candida. If you don't have bowel problems, eat cooked fruit such as a baked apple or canned, unsweetened peaches when you absolutely must have a treat.
- Fluids are very important. Make sure you drink at least 32 to 48 ounces (four to six cups) of filtered water a day and eliminate all sodas and ice-cold caffeinated teas.

Qi Gong Exercise and Meditation

Qi Gong exercise and meditation gives people in recovery an opportunity to become reacquainted with their ability to be disciplined and focused and to find a place in themselves that is free of anger and conflict. In addition, the Qi Gong breathing routines open up the Lungs and help the body let go of held-in anxiety and tension.

PROGRAM FOURTEEN: GIRLS' AND WOMEN'S HIV-RELATED PROBLEMS

The rate of increase in HIV infection among women in the United States now far exceeds that of homosexual and heterosexual men. And women are increasingly vulnerable as they are imperiled by the triple threat of drug use, sex with those who use drugs, and sex with those who practice unsafe sex.

As dependent spouses who are too often expected to be available for sexual intercourse, no questions asked, and who are not comfortable with insisting on or even allowed to insist on the use of a condom in marital relations, women are vulnerable to HIV in the same way they are vulnerable to domestic violence, rape, and other exercises of dominance by men, or in the case of lesbians, incidences of woman-to-woman violence.

For women, prevention must start with learning how to assert their self-interests and right of self-protection. This must be coupled with programs that support drug-dependent women, allow them to get off drugs without threatening their custody of their children, and protect them from violence at the hands of drug-dependent partners.

Personal responsibility for the risk of contracting HIV infection and then spreading it is essential, and women must be shown that if they are willing to do the hard work it takes to avoid exposure, society will support, not penalize, them for their efforts.

Among young women and adolescents there must be a campaign to increase their self-esteem and reinforce their ability to resist peer pressure and to resist the impulse to please men by taking unwise risks with their health. In addition, sketchy evidence of woman-to-woman transmission of HIV means that young lesbian girls must be made aware that they are not immune to the risk, either. The feeling of immortality that afflicts all teens coupled with the feelings of powerlessness and lack of self-worth that are epidemic among young girls makes this a particularly difficult task.

The confluence of psychosocial factors results in women obtaining treatment later in their development of HIV/AIDS than men and in receiving less aggressive treatment, as well. In light of HIV-positive women's increased susceptibility to breast and cervical cancer, cervical and anal dysplasia, and menstrual problems related to hormone fluctuations, it is especially important that women have access to and are encouraged to use all HIV-related health facilities and programs in their communities.

This section outlines those risks and presents a brief look at the available Chinese medicine treatments. For more detail on these issues contact one of the resource centers in Appendix 4.

PROGRAM FOR BREAST HEALTH

This four-step program combining Western and Chinese preventive and diagnostic techniques offers a simple model for women to follow that may help increase their chance of early diagnosis and treatment for breast cancer.

Step 1

Make sure to do breast self-exams monthly to look for changes in texture, shape, and color of the skin and evidence of discharge from the nipples. The American Cancer Society suggests that breast self-exams be done so that you examine the side of each breast, then the front. And make sure to palpate the area around the armpit. For complete instructions you can obtain an illustrated pamphlet from your local American Cancer Society chapter.

Step 2

Because unusual forms of breast cancer appear in HIV-positive women, regardless of your age you may want to have a baseline mammogram and then follow up every year (or more frequently, if recommended by your practitioner) with a mammogram or a mammogram and sonogram.

Step 3

Strengthen your resistance with dietary, exercise, and meditation practices. Recent studies indicate that a low-fat diet and regular exercise help protect against breast cancer. Following a natural grain- and vegetable-based diet is recommended. Regular aerobic exercise—at least 120 minutes a week, according to the American Heart Association—is also advised when possible. Daily Qi Gong meditation and breathing exercises (see Chapter 9), so essential for managing stress and keeping Qi flowing smoothly, may also help support the immune system and offer added protection.

Step 4

Preventive herbal therapy that boosts immune strength and helps stabilize hormonal fluctuations may prove beneficial. In addition to Enhance or Tremella American Ginseng, which provide basic immune system support, you may want to use Woman's Balance and Two Immortals.

PROGRAM FOR MENSTRUAL CHANGES

Women with HIV often experience changes in their menstrual cycle, including excessive bleeding, cramps, PMS, and missed periods. In addition, they are susceptible to more frequent vaginal yeast infections and to pelvic inflammatory disease. Clearly, regular medical checkups are an important part of managing these conditions. In addition, Chinese medicine offers supportive treatments that are often able to help alleviate such problems.

Herbs
In addition to Enhance or Tremella American Ginseng, your practitioner may prescribe Woman's Balance, Long Dan Xie Gan Wan, Clear Heat, or Ecliptex.

Acupuncture
For cramps and PMS—Spleen 6; Ren 4, 6; Ear Zi Gong (uterus). With Liver Qi Stagnation: Liver 3, Large Intestine 4.

For missed periods (amenorrhea)—With Xue Deficiency: Urinary Bladder 18, 20, 23; Stomach 25, 36; Spleen 6. You may also apply moxibustion to these points. With Xue Stagnation: Spleen 6, 10; Large Intestine 4, 11; Stomach 25.

Moxibustion
For general gynecological health, moxa the maintenance centers on Ren 6 and Spleen 6 plus back points along the Urinary Bladder, at Urinary Bladder 20 and 23 and the sacrum or lower back. (For the points see pages 96–102.)

For spotting—Use moxibustion on Spleen 1, Du 20, Ren 4, and Liver 1.

Diet
In addition to the diet guidelines in the basic program, following these guidelines may eliminate some of the bothersome symptoms of hormonal imbalance.

Avoid cold and raw foods, excess dairy products, all caffeine and alcohol, artificial stimulants, excess salt to avoid bloating.

Include warm, cooked, low-fat foods; increase the amount of grains and fiber you eat. Add foods rich in phytoestrogens, such as soy products, linseed oil, and red clover sprouts. Drink 48 to 64 ounces (six to eight cups) of filtered water a day.

Exercise
You can help regulate the flow of Qi and remove the stress associated with cycle-related symptoms such as PMS and menopause by a daily routine that includes Qi Gong warm-up exercises (pages 110–111) and simply walking for 20 minutes at as brisk a pace as is comfortable. Resistance training or weight lifting is probably not a great idea, however, since it can lead to a Xue deficiency and that may only increase your symptoms.

Massage

Regular professional and self-massage can help ease stress and make the discomfort easier to handle. The abdominal self-massage on page 120 is a good place to start—it helps dispel stagnation and dampness.

Reflexology on hands and feet is also highly effective in relieving tension and discomfort. See diagrams on pages 122 and 123.

PROGRAM FOR CERVICAL DYSPLASIA

Women who are HIV-positive are at considerably higher risk for cervical dysplasia—also called cervical intraepithelial neoplasia, or CIN—an abnormality of the squamous cells that line the cervix and in some cases may be a precursor of cervical cancer. In fact, Pap tests of HIV-positive women reveal abnormalities in almost 50 percent tested and more detailed examination with colposcopy detects abnormalities in 87 percent of the tests. This dramatic finding may be related to the higher incidence of infection with the sexually transmitted disease called human papilloma virus (HPV). Certain strains of HPV are highly associated with the development of cervical cancer and it appears that those who are HIV-positive may be more susceptible to those strains and those strains may have a stronger negative effect on the cervix. But whatever the cause, the higher rate of abnormal cervical cells makes vigilance vitally important. To aid in prompt diagnosis most doctors recommend a Pap test every six months for all women who are HIV-positive, regardless of age.

Chinese treatments center around herbal formulas and acupuncture and have proved highly effective in reversing some early stages of cervical dysplasia. Men—and women—with anal dysplasia can also follow this program.

Herbs

The herbal formulas recommended include Clear Heat, Isatis Cooling, Liu Wei Di Huang Wan, Shen Gem.

Acupuncture and Moxibustion

If you have an abnormal Pap test, you may want to begin treatments once a week until your next Pap test.

- General acupuncture for dysplasia—Ren 2; Stomach 30, Ba Liao, Zi Gong (uterus), and Ear Zi Gong.
- For Kidney and Liver Yin Deficiency—Kidney 3, 6, 7; Lung 7; Urinary Bladder 18, 23; Spleen 6; Ren 6; Ear Kidney; Ear Liver.
- For Heat in the Lower Triple Burner—Liver 2, 5; Urinary Bladder 57; and Du 1.

- For Spleen Qi Deficiency—Stomach 36, Spleen 6, Urinary Bladder 20, Ren 12, Liver 13. Moxibustion on all those points twice a week.
- For Damp Heat in the Liver channel—Liver 2, 5; Spleen 9; Gallbladder 27; Stomach 30; Ren 3, 4; Ear Gallbladder; Ear Liver.

When a chapter in one's life ends, and the next is not yet started, there is an opportunity for reflection. As you come to the end of this book, I hope that you will take time to look back at its central message: You are in charge of your healing process and you can do a great deal to improve the quality of your daily life. Although I was not able to cover every aspect of HIV-related diseases and disorders—particularly the problems of diabetes, prostate problems in men, and the special challenges facing HIV-positive adolescents and children—it is my most cherished hope that you will find this book provides you with the knowledge you need to empower your mind/body/spirit.

Notes

Chapter 1—In Honor of Those Living with HIV/AIDS

1. D. Abrams, *Alternative Therapies in HIV Infection, AIDS* (1990): 1179–1187; D. I. Abrams, "Alternative Therapies," in N. P. Repoza, ed., *HIV Infection and Disease* (Chicago: A.M.A. Press, 1989), 163–175.

Chapter 4—Toxic Heat Spleen/Stomach Deficiency, and the Human Immunodeficiency Virus: HIV Disease from the Chinese Perspective

1. D. I. Abrams, "Dealing with Alternative Therapies for HIV," in M. A. Sande and P. A. Volberding, eds., *The Medical Management of AIDS*, 4th ed. (Philadelphia: W. B. Saunders, 1995), 183–207; Qingcai Zhang, M.D., and Hong-Yen Hsu, Ph.D., *AIDS and Chinese Medicine* (New Canaan, Conn.: Keats Publishing, 1995).

Chapter 5—The War Within: Western Immunology and HIV

In Figure 2, The Cellular Processes Impacted by Various Antiviral Medications, Antiviral medicines may prevent the replication of the HIV virus in several ways. Some, such as those listed in the first column of the illustration on page 43 under soluble CD4, may block the virus by preventing it from penetrating potential host cells. Others, such as the nucleoside analogs (AZT and 3TC); nucleotide analogs; and nonneucleoside reverse transcriptase (RT) inhibitors (delavirdine [U90] and nevirapine [BI-RG-587], and efivirens [DMP 266], for example, work by inhibiting the essential action of the enzyme reverse transcriptase in the replication process or by interfering with the successful production of complementary viral DNA chains. Interferons and some other drugs work on yet another process: They keep the replicated HIV virus inside the host cell from being fully developed. Protease inhibitors, interferons, and glycosylation inhibitors prevent assembly and release of the virus.

1. Ronald A. Barker, Mackewicz, and Levy, *PNAS* 92 (1995): 1135.

2. Y. Cao, L. Qin, L. Zhang, J. Safrit, D. D. Ho, "Virologic and Immunologic Characterization of Long-Term Survivors of Human Immunodeficiency Virus Type 1 Infection," *New England Journal of Medicine* 332, 4 (Jan. 26, 1995): 201–208.

3. G. Pantaleo et al., "Studies in Subjects with Long-Term Nonprogressive Human

Immunodeficiency Virus Infection," *New England Journal of Medicine* 332, 4 (Jan. 26, 1995): 209–216.

4. *New England Journal of Medicine* 334 (1996): 1065–1066.

Chapter 6—Nurturing the Mind/Body/Spirit: The HIV + Dietary Program

1. Kathleen Mulligan et al., "Anabolic Effects of Recombinant Human Growth Hormone in Patients with Wasting Associated with Human Immunodeficiency Virus Infection," *Journal of Clinical Endocrinology and Metabolism* 77, 1 (1993).

2. John P. Palenicek et al., "Weight Loss Prior to Clinical AIDS as a Predictor of Survival," *Journal of Acquired Immune Deficiency Syndromes and Human Retrovirology* 10, 3 (1995).

3. Mulligan, op. cit.

4. Ulrich Suttmann et al., "Incidence and Prognostic Value of Malnutrition and Wasting in Human Immunodeficiency Virus–Infected Patients," *Journal of Acquired Immune Deficiency Syndromes and Human Retrovirology* 8, 3 (1995).

5. Mary Romeyn, M.D., *Nutrition and HIV: A New Model for Treatment* (San Francisco: Jossey-Bass Publishers, 1995).

6. D. A. Fryburg et al., "The Immunostimulatory Effects and Safety of Beta-carotene in Patients with AIDS," presented at the Eighth International Conference on AIDS, Amsterdam, July 19–24, 1992.

7. A. M. Tang et al., "Low Serum Vitamin B12 Concentrations Are Associated with Faster Human Immunodeficiency Virus Type 1 (HIV-1) Disease Progression," *Journal of Nutrition* 127, 2 (1997): 345–351.

8. G. Shor-Posner et al., "Impact of Vitamin B6 Status on Psychological Distress in a Longitudinal Study of HIV-1 Infection," *International Journal of Psychiatry and Medicine* 24, 3 (1994): 209–222.

9. A. R. Berger et al., "Dose Response, Coasting, and Differential Fiber Vulnerability in Human Toxic Neuropathy: A Prospective Study of Pyridoxine Neurotoxicity," *Neurology* 42, 7 (1992): 1367–1370; J. A. Waterston and B. S. Gilligan, "Pyridoxine Neuropathy," *Medical Journal of Australia* 146, 12 (1987): 640–642; G. J. Parry and D. E. Bredesen, "Sensory Neuropathy with Low-Dose Pyridoxine," *Neurology* 35, 10 (1985): 1466–1468.

10. R. Kinscherf et al., "Effect of Glutathione Depletion and Oral N-acetyl-cysteine Treatment on CD4+ and CD8+ Cells," *FASEB J* 8, 6 (1994): 448–451; J. S. James, "NAC: First Controlled Trial, Positive Results," *AIDS Treatment News*, no. 250 (July 5, 1996): 1.

Chapter 7—The Basic HIV + Herbal Therapy Program: Prescription for Enhanced Balance and Strength

1. H. Yeung, *Handbook of Chinese Herbs and Formulas* (1985).

2. Selway, *Plant Flavonoids in Biology and Medicine* (1986).

3. *Cancer* 52 (1983): 70–73.

4. Cancer Institute of the Chinese Academy of Medical Sciences, "Astragalus Update," *Professional Health Concerns* 102 (1988): 2.

5. Minxing Zhou et al., "Therapeutic Effect of Astragalus in Treating Chronic Active Hepatitis and the Changes in Immune Functions," *Journal of Chinese People's Liberation Army* 7, 4 (1982): 242–244.

6. *Chinese Medical Journal* 94, 1 (1981): 35–40.

7. Ibid.

8. H.-Y. Hsu, *Oriental Materia Medica: A Concise Guide* (San Francisco: Oriental Healing Arts Institute, 1986), 523.

9. Yeung, op. cit., 293.

10. *Methods and Findings in Experimental and Clinical Pharmacology* 9 (Nov. 14, 1992): 725–736.

11. Yeung, op. cit., 89.

12. S. Dharmananda, private conversation.

13. Terry Willard, *Reishi Mushroom: Herb of Spiritual Potency and Medical Wonder* (Port Jervis, N.Y.: Lubrecht & Cramer, 1995), 12.

14. Takashi, *Chemistry Abstracts* 98: 212585t; Hsu, op. cit., 641; *Becoming Healthy with Reishi*, III, 1988, 12–20.

15. *Chemistry Abstracts* 93: 542y.

16. *Pharmacology and Applications of Chinese Materia Medica* (1986): 642–653.

17. *Chemistry Abstracts* 92: 51937t.

18. *Becoming Healthy with Reishi*, III, 1988, 12–20.

19. Willard, op. cit.

20. *Chemical and Pharmaceutical Bulletin* 36, 6 (1988): 2090–2097.

21. *Chung-Kuo* 13, 3 (1993): 147–149.

22. *Fortschritte der Medizin* 110, 21 (1992): 395–398.

23. Hsu, op. cit., 590.

24. R. S. Chang and H. W. Yeung, *Antiviral Research* 9 (1988): 163.

25. Bensky and Gamble, *Chinese Materia Medica*, rev. ed. (Seattle: Eastland Press, 1993), 378.

26. Yeung, *Handbook of Chinese Herbs and Formulas*, 93.

27. *Bulletin of the World Health Organization* 67, 6 (1989): 613–680.

28. Hsu, op. cit., 243.

29. Bensky and Gamble, op. cit., 91.

30. Hsu, op. cit., 470.

31. Bensky and Gamble, op. cit., 269.

32. Yeung, op. cit., 125.

33. H. F. Chiu et al., "Pharmacological and Pathological Studies on Hepatic Protective Crude Drugs from Taiwan," *American Journal of Chinese Medicine* 20, 3–4 (1992): 257–264.

34. Bensky and Gamble, op. cit., 365.

35. J. J. Carter, "Liver Protection and Repair: Synthesizing Herbal Science and Chinese Energetics," *Professional Health Concerns* 3, 1: 21–24.

36. Ibid.

37. Ibid.

Appendix 1:

A Personal Journey through Landmarks and Highlights in Chinese Medicine and HIV/AIDS Treatment in the United States

The following is my personal view of the development of the treatment of HIV/AIDS using Chinese medicine. Although it has a strong focus on major influences on the evolution of the Quan Yin Healing Arts Center and Chicken Soup Chinese Medicine protocols for treatment of HIV/AIDS, I want to acknowledge all the people and programs who have contributed to the overall development of treatment of HIV/AIDS using Chinese medicine in the United States. Not everyone could be mentioned in this list owing to the large number of people and organizations involved.

219
  • *Shang Han Lun (Treatise on Cold-Induced Febrile Disease)* by Zhang Zhong Jing—a landmark book on herbal medicine for epidemic disease, used throughout the world today.

1798
  • *Wen Bing Tiao Ben (Detailed Analysis of Epidemic Febrile Disease)* published by Wu Tang—a landmark book on warm epidemic disease

1970s
  • Fu Zheng Therapy Coordinating Group, a research organization in China, begins to work with cancer therapies based on Fu Zheng (Support the Normal, or immunotherapy) to support the body during chemotherapy treatment for cancer.

1981
  • International conference held in Harbin, China, cosponsored by the Academy of Traditional Medicine (Beijing) and the University of Texas Health Sciences Center, attended by Subhuti Dharmananda, Ph.D., of the Institute

for Traditional Medicine (ITM). The first time word goes out from China about Fu Zheng research.

1982–83

• Lincoln Detox Acupuncture Clinic in the South Bronx begins treating people with AIDS/ARC (AIDS-related complex) with acupuncture under the direction of Michael O. Smith, M.D. In 1989, Lincoln Detox begins to use herbal formulas provided by Angela Shen, O.M.D.

1983

• Human Immunodeficiency Virus (HIV) identified at the Pasteur Institute in Paris.

1984

• Quan Yin Acupuncture and Herb Center, cofounded by Misha Cohen, O.M.D., L.Ac., with Cindy Icke, O.M.D., L.Ac., opens its doors in San Francisco and begins treating people with HIV/AIDS with full-service Chinese medicine treatments.

1985

• Reece Smith, L.Ac., and Subhuti Dharmananda, Ph.D., publish "AIDS Prevention: Considerations on the Management of the Prodrome Symptoms Using the Concept of Traditional Chinese Medicine" in the *Journal of the American College of Traditional Chinese Medicine*. Article outlines a model for understanding HIV in terms of Chinese medicine.

• The San Francisco AIDS Alternative Healing Project (SFAAHP) is founded by Quan Yin Acupuncture and Herb Center and AIDS activists. SFAAHP provided comprehensive healing programs from 1985 until it closed in 1990.

1986

• AZT is released, and Chinese medicine practitioners begin treating side effects of Western antiviral drugs with Chinese medicine. We had been treating side effects of medications for opportunistic infections prior to this.

• Astra Eight, an herbal formula for general immune deficiency, is designed by Subhuti Dharmamanda, Ph.D.

• Immune Enhancement Program in Berkeley studies 20 people with ARC using Astra Eight formula under the direction of Susan Black, R.N. Improvements are noted, especially the ability of severely ill people to return to work. Quan Yin begins using this formula in pill and cooked form, and results are resoundingly better than with earlier herbal formulas. Astra Eight is composed mostly of Qi tonic herbs.

• *Living with AIDS: Reaching Out*, by Tom O'Connor with Ahmed Gonzalez-Nunez, published. This book covered the gamut of alternative therapies as used in a comprehensive approach, including "The Use of Herbs in AIDS and ARC" by Dr. Cohen. This book was used extensively at Quan Yin as a guide to natural therapies.

• *Psychoimmunity and the Healing Process: A Holistic Approach to Immunity and AIDS*, by Jason Serinus, is published. This book includes information on Chinese medicine, with Dr. Cohen providing input.

1987

• World Congress of Acupuncture and Natural Medicine, Beijing, China, includes some of first presentations in China on AIDS by Michael O. Smith, M.D., and Misha Cohen, O.M.D.

• Astra 10 Plus and Viola 12 are developed by Dr. Dharmananda. They produce improved results—people with HIV infection can take herbs over a long period of time without becoming too congested or overheated or having as many digestive complaints.

• AIDS Alternative Healing Project in Chicago treats 84 people with AIDS with acupuncture under direction of Pam Mills, certified acupuncturist.

• "Acupuncture and the AIDS Epidemic: Reflections on the Treatment of 200 Patients in Four Years," by Naomi Rabinowitz, M.D., published in the *American Journal of Acupuncture*. Describes treatment of AIDS at Lincoln Detox Acupuncture Clinic in the South Bronx.

• Dr. Cohen, working with the SFAAHP, joins Dr. Dharmananda to form a program to test herbal formulas in people with HIV and CFIDS (chronic fatigue immune deficiency syndrome). This leads to the collaboration from 1987 to 1988 with Dr. Qingcai Zhang and the Oriental Healing Arts Institute, supported by the Brion Herb Corporation and BioHerb, Inc.

• The Austin (Texas) Immune Clinic begins treatment of people with AIDS using Chinese medicine, under the direction of Brian McKenna and Carla Wilson, L.Ac. An observational study is undertaken in cooperation with the University of Texas Nursing School.

1988

• The Ninth Annual Symposium of the Oriental Healing Arts Institute, Long Beach, California, "AIDS, Immunity, and Chinese Medicine." Presentations on HIV/AIDS include those by Qingcai Zhang, M.D.; Subhuti Dharmananda, Ph.D.; Michael O. Smith, M.D.; Keith Barton, M.D.; and Misha Cohen, O.M.D. Dr. Qingcai Zhang presents results of the SFAAHP herbal program at this symposium.

• "Results of Chinese Medical Treatment Show Frequent Symptom Relief and Some Apparent Long-Term Remission," by Michael O. Smith, M.D., published in the *American Journal of Acupuncture*. It is a summary of work to date at Lincoln Detox Acupuncture Clinic.

• Quan Yin Healing Arts Center, the nonprofit arm of Quan Yin Acupuncture and Herb Center, expands treatment of HIV-positive clients, initiating the Quan Yin Herbal Program for HIV-positive People, with support from ITM.

• Dr. Chang of the University of California–Davis and Dr. Yeung of Hong Kong identify 11 Chinese herbs as antiviral or virucidal against HIV in vitro (*Antiviral Research* 9 [1988]: 163–176).

1989

• Dr. Wei Bei Hai, visiting professor from Beijing College of Traditional Chinese Medicine, proposes theory of Spleen/Stomach disorders as primary in HIV/AIDS at Quan Yin Healing Arts Center–sponsored symposium.

1989–90

• The Healthshare Project of the Portland Addictions Center begins to offer full-service Chinese and naturopathic medicine to people with HIV under the direction of David Eisen, L.Ac., MSW, OMD.

1989–90

• Composition A and Composition herbal formulas, designed by Subhuti Dharmananda of ITM, the first formulas designed specifically for people with HIV, are tested at the Quan Yin Herbal Program for HIV-positive People.

1990

• Quan Yin Acupuncture and Herb Center closes after San Francisco Loma Prieta earthquake; Quan Yin Healing Arts Center (with initial support from a benefactor) remains open and committed to treating people with HIV/AIDS.

• Completion of the Quan Yin Herbal Program for HIV-positive People. Over 600 HIV-positive clients are enrolled in 1988–90.

• El Rio, a cutting-edge comprehensive addiction-treatment program based on alternatives to incarceration, is founded by Ana Oliveira, L.Ac., as part of the Osborne Association in the South Bronx. The program includes acupuncture for substance abuse. In 1992, Carla Wilson, L.Ac., begins a full-service Chinese medicine clinic, Clinica El Rio de la Vida, which serves HIV-infected people in the South Bronx, including acupuncture.

• The Quan Yin Professional HIV Certification Program is designed by Katharine Woodruff, R.N., and Dr. Cohen, with startup funding from Colin Higgins and Horizons Foundations. The program continues to provide state-of-the-art East-West education for Chinese medicine practitioners. As of 1996, more than 250 practitioners worldwide, including M.D.s, have taken the course.

• "Chinese Medicine in the Treatment of Chronic Immunodeficiency: Diagnosis and Treatment," by Misha Cohen, is published in the *American Journal of Acupuncture*.

• The Immune Enhancement Program (IEP) is formed in San Francisco. The current director is Thomas Sinclair, L.Ac.

1991

• The International Symposium on Viral Hepatitis and AIDS is held in Beijing, China. "Development of Herbal Treatment Protocols for HIV Infection and Other Chronic Viral Diseases" is presented by Dr. Cohen, as well as results of the Quan Yin Herbal Program for HIV-positive people.

1991–present

• Dr. Cohen develops herbal formulas that are now used internationally by Chinese medicine practitioners for the treatment of HIV/AIDS: 1991–1994—Enhance and Clear Heat; 1992—Marrow Plus; 1994–Source Qi and Tremella American Ginseng.

1992

• The Center for Disease Control issues a new definition of AIDS based on a CD4+ count below 200.

• Publication of *The Treatment of AIDS and Chinese Medicine,* by Dr. Huang Bing Shan, based on observational studies at the Austin (Texas) Immune Clinic.

• Publication of *Treatment of AIDS with Traditional Chinese Medicine,* translated by Wang Qi Lang (Shandong Science and Technology Press).

• Double-blind study funded by the University of California–San Francisco and conducted at San Francisco General Hospital on the application of Chinese herbal therapies for HIV disease. Jeff Burack, principal investigator, with Misha Cohen, O.M.D.; Donald Abrams, M.D., professor of medicine and director of San Francisco Community Consortium; and Judith Hahn, M.S. The study includes San Francisco General Hospital, Quan Yin Healing Arts Center, and the University of California–San Francisco.

• The first Chinese medicine clinics are funded by CARE (Ryan White) Funds for direct care to people with HIV/AIDS; the first two are: Immune Enhancement Project (IEP) and the American College of Traditional Chinese Medicine under the Alternative Health Category.

1993

• The International AIDS Symposium in Berlin breaks new ground by including an official presentation on HIV and Chinese and alternative therapies, including a presentation by Donald Abrams, M.D.; David Baker, M.S.N., R.N.; and Misha Cohen, O.M.D.

Poster presentation of San Francisco General Hospital "Herbal Therapies for HIV Disease," highlighting important collaborative work between Chinese medicine and Western practitioners; J. Burack, M. Cohen, D. Abrams, J. Hahn.

Poster presentation on Chinese herbal observational treatment at the IEP by David Baker, R.N.

- The First International HIV/AIDS and Chinese Medicine Conference held at San Francisco State University.
- *Treating AIDS with Chinese Medicine,* by Mary Kay Ryan and Arthur D. Shattuck, is published. They put forth a different view from the Spleen/Stomach analysis of HIV infection.

1993–97

Government- and university-sponsored Chinese medicine studies begun and/or funded:

- Donald I. Abrams, M.D., principal investigator; Misha Cohen, O.M.D., coinvestigator.

Treatment of HIV-Related Anemia with Chinese Herbs. Conducted by the Community Consortium; funded by the NIH. To be completed in 1998.

- Donald I. Abrams, M.D., principal investigator; Misha Cohen, O.M.D., coinvestigator.

Chinese Herbal Treatment for HIV-Related Diarrhea. Conducted by the Community Consortium; funded by University of California–San Francisco. To be completed in 1998.

- Rainer Weber, M.D., principal investigator; Misha Cohen, O.M.D., Silvio Schaller, Prak. Arzt, coinvestigators.

Chinese Herbal Treatment for HIV-related Symptoms. Funded by the Swiss National Foundation for AIDS Research. Study to be completed 1998.

- Tom Sinclair, L.Ac., principal investigator.

Immune Enhancement Program study of sinusitis, funded by the NIH's Office of Alternative Medicine.

- Leanna Standish, N.D., principal investigator.

In 1994, Bastyr University in Seattle is funded by the NIH's Office of Alternative Medicine to establish the AIDS Research Center. The purpose of the center is to conduct a nationwide study on the use of alternative/complementary therapies for the treatment of HIV/AIDS.
Other studies:

- Acupuncture and Elavil. This NIH trial is looking at acupuncture and Elavil (amitriptyline) for the treatment of peripheral neuropathy.

1994

- The Second International HIV/AIDS and Chinese Medicine Conference sponsored by the newly formed AIDS and Chinese Medicine Institute (ACMI) is held at San Francisco State University.
- "Using Acupuncture and Herbs for the Treatment of HIV Infection: The American College of Traditional Chinese Medicine Experience," by Howard Moffet et al., is published in *AIDS Patient Care.*

1994–present

• A study of acupuncture in the treatment of HIV-related chronic hepatitis is begun with Misha Cohen as principal investigator. It is conducted by Quan Yin Healing Arts and funded by the Thomas O'Connor Foundation.

1995

• In a groundbreaking meeting of East and West, an NIH-sponsored ad hoc meeting on the use of alternative medicine in the treatment of people with HIV/AIDS assembles a panel to discuss the benefits and dangers of complementary and alternative medicine that includes Wayne Jonas, M.D., cochair and director, Office of Alternative Medicine, NIH; Kiyoshi Kuromiya, cochair, Critical Path Project, NIH AIDS Evaluation Working Group; Donald Abrams, M.D., professor of medicine at University of California–San Francisco and assistant director, AIDS Program at San Francisco General Hospital; Ronald Baker, Ph.D., director, Treatment Education and Advocacy, San Francisco AIDS Foundation; Carola Burroughs, Holistic Connections; Misha Cohen, O.M.D., research and education director, Quan Yin Healing Arts Center; Leonard Herzenberg, Ph.D., professor of genetics, Stanford University; John James, publisher of *AIDS Treatment News*; and Michael Onstott, community activist.

• The Third International HIV/AIDS and Chinese Medicine Conference is held at Columbia University.

1996

• The Fourth International HIV/AIDS and Chinese Medicine Conference is held in Los Angeles.

• Quan Yin Healing Arts Center receives CARE (Ryan White) funds under the Primary Care Category for Chinese medicine care. Now five Chinese medicine programs in San Francisco as well as other programs around the country are funded by CARE.

1997

• Protease inhibitors and triple-combination therapy are established as Western standard of treatment. This powerful medicine requires additional Chinese medicine treatment of increased side effects.

Appendix 2:

Quan Yin Herbal Program–
Sample Formula Guide

These formulas are intended to be used only when prescribed by a practitioner and should not be bought over-the-counter or used without ongoing medical supervision. For information about ingredients, have your practitioner contact the manufacturer.

Formula and Company	Actions	Typical Applications
Enhance (Health Concerns)	Tonification Clear Heat Clean toxin Vitalize Regulate Qi and Xue	Chronic viral infections Immune deficiency
Tremella American Ginseng (Health Concerns)	Tonify Yin Clear Heat Clean toxin Vitalize Regulate Qi and Xue	Chronic viral infections Immune deficiency
Clear Heat (Health Concerns)	Clear Heat Remove toxins	Infections HIV bone marrow infections
Marrow Plus (Health Concerns)	Tonify/vitalize blood	Drug toxicity Anemia Decreased white and red blood cell counts
Source Qi (Health Concerns)	Tonify and warm Spleen and Stomach Systems	Chronic diarrhea
Ecliptex (Health Concerns)	Regulate Qi Vitalize blood	Chronic hepatitis Impaired liver function
Allereze (Karuna)	Warm Lung Diaphoretic	Bronchial asthma allergies

Formula and Company	Actions	Typical Applications
Clear Air (Health Concerns)	Clear Toxic Heat Stop cough Cold/damp	Acute upper respiratory infection
Zhi Sou Ding Chuan Wan	Stop cough Relieve asthma	Acute asthma symptoms
Phellostatin (Health Concerns)	Clear Heat and damp	Candidiasis Intestinal yeast Fatigue Bloating
Artestatin (Health Concerns)	Remove parasites Diarrhea	Intestinal parasites Giardia
Aquilaria 22 (7 Forests)	Remove parasites Astringe intestines	Chronic parasites with constipation
Coptis Purge Fire (Health Concerns)	Remove Damp Heat	Herpes infection Ear/sinus/throat infections
Lung Tan Xie Gan Wan	Remove Damp Heat	Herpes infection Ear/sinus/throat infections
Laminaria 4 (Health Concerns)	Resolve heated phlegm	Lymph swelling Resolve nodules
Li Gan Pian (Liver-strengthening tablets) (Zheng Jiang)	Dredge liver	Liver inflammation Increased enzymes
CMV Retinitis* Formula	Clear Heat Toxin	Cytomegalovirus retinitis
Schizandra Dreams (Health Concerns)	Nourish heart	Insomnia Palpitations Emotional instability Night sweats
Isatis Cooling (Health Concerns)	Clear Heat Remove Dampness	Vaginal infections Yellow discharges Urinary tract infection
Chin-Chiu and Tortoise Shell (Brion Herb Corporation)	Tonify Yin	MAC Tuberculosis without cough
Yun Nan Pai Yao	Stop bleeding	Hemorrhaging Acute injury Bleeding
Zaocys Tablets (Seven Forests)	Remove surface heat	Chronic itching

*Practitioners: E-mail TCMpaths@aol.com for formula, not product

Formula and Company	Actions	Typical Applications
Kochia 13 (Seven Forests)	Remove surface heat Stop itching	Chronic itching
Woman's Balance (Health Concerns)	Tonify Spleen and Xue Regulate Liver Qi	PMS Chronic hepatitis Dysmenorrhea
Vagistatin (Health Concerns)	Remove Dampness/Heat	Vaginitis Vaginal candidiasis
Two Immortals (Health Concerns)	Tonify Liver and Kidney Yin	Menopausal symptoms Hot flashes Night sweats

Appendix 3:

The Medicine Cabinet

There are a few herbal formulas that you can keep on hand at home to take as needed when specific symptoms arise. The following products are generally available at health food stores and at alternative health centers. The ingredients are given here so that you and your practitioner may check for any interactions between formulas you are taking.

Formula and Company	Actions	Ingredients	
Cold Free One (Pacific Biologics)	Eliminate exogenous pathogen *Typical Application:* Common cold/ influenza	Each tablet contains: Honeysuckle Great Burdock Reed Rhizome Forsythia Balloon Flower Ning Po Figwort Mulberry Root	Bamboo Leaves Chrysanthemum Soybean Schizonepeta Peppermint Licorice Root
Yin Chiao Chieh Tu Pien (Beijing Tung Jin)	Eliminate exogenous pathogen *Typical Application:* Common cold/ influenza	*Each tablet contains:* Jin Yin Hua Lian Qiao Niu Bang Zi Jie Geng Bo He Lu Gen Gan Cao Dan Zhu Ye Jing Jie	Lonicera Flower Forsythia Fruit Arctii Lappa Fruit Radix Platycodi Herba Menthae Rhizome Phragmites Radix Glycyrrhiza Herba Lopatheri Schizonepeta Flower
Isatis Gold (Health Concerns)	Eliminate exogenous pathogen *Typical Application:* Common cold/ influenza	*Each tablet contains:* Echinacea Goldenseal Ligusticum Platycodon Isatis extract	*Echinacea purpurea* *Hydrastis canadensis* Chuan Xiong Jie Geng Ban Lan Gen and Da Qing Ye
Pe Min Kan Wan (Plum Flower)	Open surface Clear blocked sinuses	*Each tablet contains:* Cang Er Zi Huo Xiang	Xanthium Fruit Herba Agastache

Formula and Company	Actions	Ingredients	
	Typical Application: Chronic/acute sinusitis	Ju Hua Bai Zhi Xin Yin Hua Jin Yin Hua	Chrysanthemum Angelica Dahurica Magnolia Flower Honeysuckle
San She Dan (United Pharmacies)	Stop cough Clear Damp *Typical Application:* Cough with green-yellow or dry phlegm	*Always contains:* She Dan Chen Pi Snake Bile	 Agkistrodon Acutus Pericarpium Citri Reticulatae
Loquat Extract (Nin Jiom)	Stop cough *Typical Application:* Cough	*Each tablet contains:* Pi Pa Ye Ban Xia Bei Mu Bo He Sha Shen Kuan Dong Hua Wu Wei Zi Xing Ren Chen Pi Feng Mi Jie Geng	 Fol. Eriobotryae Japonicae Rz. Pinelliae Ternatae Bulbus Fritillariae Herba Menthae Rx. Glehniae Littoralis Tussilagi Farfarae Flower Schizandrae Chinensis Fruit Semen Pruni Armenicae Pericarpium Citri Reticulatae Honey Rx. Platycodi Grandiflori
Quiet Digestion (Health Concerns)	Increase Spleen/ Stomach function *Typical Application:* Difficult digestion Distention Nausea	*Each tablet contains:* Fu Ling Huo Xiang Yi Yi Ren Gu Ya Shen Chu Tian Hua Fen Hou Po Ju Hua Bai Zhi Chi Shi Zhi Ge Gen	 Poria Pogostemon Coix Oryza Shen Qu Trichosanthes Magnolia Chrysanthemum Angelica Halloysite Pueraria

Formula and Company	Actions	Ingredients	
		Ju Hong	Citrus
		Cang Zhu	Red Atractylodes
		Bo He	Herba Menthae
		Mu Xiang	Saussurea
		Malt	
Pill Curing (Kang Ning Wan)	Increase Spleen/ Stomach function	*Each tablet contains:* Tian Ma	Rz. Gastrodiae Elatae
	Typical Application: Difficult digestion Distention Nausea	Bai Zhi	Rx. Angelicae
		Ju Hua	Fl. Chrysanthemum
		Bo He	Herba Menthae
		Ge Gen	Rx. Puerariae
		Tian Hua Fen	Rx. Trichosanthes
		Cang Zhu	Rz. Atractylodes
		Yi Mi	S. Coicis Lachryma-jobi
		Fu Ling	Schlerotium Poria Cocos
		Mu Xiang	Rx. Saussurea
		Hou Po	Cx. Magnolia officinalis
		Ju Hong	Pericarpium Citri Erythrocarpae
		Huo Xiang	Herba Agastaches seu Pogostemi
White Flower Oil (For external use— available from Chinese herb store)	Clear sinuses	*Contains:* Wintergreen oil	
	Typical Application: Stuffy sinuses from colds, Allergies Chronic sinusitis (Use one drop in steaming water and inhale at a distance from the water's surface. Oil is strong; be careful not to burn eyes)	Menthol Camphor Some brands contain eucalyptus oil	

Appendix 4:

Resources

How to Find a Qualified Licensed Chinese Medicine Practitioner

Call or write the following organizations for referrals and certificate information.

Acupuncture.com
www.acupuncture.com
Up-to-date and complete listing of acupuncturists across the country.

National Certification Commission for Acupuncture and Oriental Medicine
1464 16th Street NW, Suite 501
Washington, DC 20036
Tel: 202-232-1404
Fax: 202-462-6157
Can provide list of nationally certified practitioners.

American Association of Oriental Medicine (AAOM)
433 Front Street
Catasauqua, PA 18032-2506
Tel: 610-266-1433
Fax: 610-264-2768
Member-practitioner organization.

National Acupuncture and Oriental Medicine Alliance (NAOMA)
14637 Starr Road SE
Olalla, WA 98359
Tel: 253-851-6896
Fax: 253-851-6883
This is a professional membership organization of acupuncturists, Asian medicine providers, and acupuncture-related organizations.

National Detoxification Association (NADA) Clearinghouse
P.O. Box 1927
Vancouver, WA 98668
Tel: 360-260-8620
NADA provides information on national and international drug and alcohol detoxification programs and trains practitioners.

Quan Yin Healing Arts Center
1748 Market Street
San Francisco, CA 94102
Tel: 415-861-4964
Fax: 415-861-0579
E-mail: QYHAC@aol.com
Carla Wilson, executive director

Quan Yin can provide a list of practitioners trained through the Quan Yin HIV Professional Certification Program. See also "Healing Centers," below.

AIDS and Chinese Medicine Institute (ACMI)
See page 218 for contact information.

ACMI provides HIV-positive people with a list of practitioners who have completed their basic HIV track at the ACMI-sponsored AIDS and Chinese Medicine Conference.

Healing Centers

The following centers provide a full range of Chinese and complementary therapies for people with HIV. You may contact them for an appointment, to arrange for a telephone consultation, or to request literature.

AIDS Alternative Health Project
4753 N. Broadway, Suite 1110
Chicago, IL 60640
Tel: 773-561-2800
Contact: Michael Brickmand, executive director

Alive & Well
540 W. Broadway
Glendale, CA 91204
Tel: 818-247-5125
Contact: Nancy Rez, R.N.

Chicken Soup Chinese Medicine
San Francisco, CA 94103
Fax: 415-864-9653
E-mail: CHINMEDSF@aol.com
Web address: www.docmisha.com
Misha Cohen, director

Misha Cohen's private clinic. All treatments by appointment only; a limited number of phone consultations are available.

Chicken Soup Chinese Medicine maintains a Web site within Channel A.com that features a virtual visit to a Chinese medicine practitioner, "Ask Doc Misha," providing answers to and advice about health issues, a women's health section, and a growing area on HIV/AIDS and Chinese medicine. You may also order this book (Holt, 1998), and *The Chinese Way to Healing: Many Paths to Wholeness* (Perigee, 1996), Dr. Cohen's book describing Chinese medicine in detail, at this Web site.

Community Health Acupuncture Network (CHAN)
HIV/AIDS Clinic Working Group
c/o Karin Hilsdale, L.Ac.
301 S. Fair Oaks, #102
Pasadena, CA 91105
Tel: 301-578-1080, ext. 218
   Provides training in the Los Angeles area for Chinese medicine practitioners.

Fenway Community Health Center
7 Haviland Street
Boston, MA 02115
Tel: 617-267-0900

Immune Enhancement Program
2009 S.E. Hawthorne Boulevard
Portland, OR 97214-3819
Tel: 503-233-2101

Immune Enhancement Project (in San Francisco)
3450 16th Street
San Francisco, CA 94114
Tel: 415-252-8711
Fax: 415-252-8710
Email: www.creative.net\~*iep*
Tom Sinclair, executive director
   Offers acupuncture, herbs, and massage for HIV-positive people.

Kang Wen Acupuncture Clinic
1111 Harvard Avenue
Seattle, WA 98122-4205
Tel: 206-322-6945

Portland Addictions Acupuncture Center
1201 S.W. Morrison Street
Portland, OR 97205-2219
Tel: 503-228-4533
David Eisen, L.Ac., M.S.W., O.M.D., director
   Full-service Chinese and naturopathic medicine to people with HIV infection.

Qingcai Zhang, M.D. (China), L.Ac.
Sino-Med Research Institute
141 East 44th Street, Suite 712
New York, NY 10017
Tel: 212-573-9584
   Dr. Zhang includes therapies such as allicin (garlic) treatment and bitter melon as part of Chinese and natural therapy treatment in his clinic.

Quan Yin Healing Arts Center
1748 Market Street, Suite 202
San Francisco, CA 94102
Tel: 415-861-4964
  Quan Yin Healing Arts Center offers in-house and phone consultations. It also offers the general public lecture series and classes, such as on Qi Gong. For practitioners, there is the Quan Yin Professional HIV Certification Program and Quan Yin Professional Education Series.

Naomi Rabinowitz, M.D.
1841 Broadway, Suite 509
New York, NY 10023
Tel: 212-489-5038
  Private practice. Was affiliated with Lincoln Detox for several years. Many years of experience with HIV and Chinese medicine—uses acupuncture and herb protocols.

Public Workshops/Classes

The following provide information and/or training in various healing arts.

Paths to Wholeness Workshops
P.O. Box 135
3128 16th Street
San Francisco, CA 94103
Tel: 415-864-7234
Fax: 415-864-9653
E-mail: TCMPaths@aol.com
  Dr. Cohen offers Paths to Wholeness Workshops for the general public and health professionals other than Chinese medicine practitioners. Workshops include:

1. Focus on HIV/AIDS
2. Focus on Women's Health
3. The Chinese Medicine Cabinet: Using Chinese Herbs for Optimum Health

  Dr. Cohen will also teach seminars on other topics upon request.

Professional Seminars/Classes

AIDS and Chinese Medicine Institute
See page 218 for contact information.

Paths to Wholeness Professional Seminars
P.O. Box 135
3128 16th Street
San Francisco, CA 94103
Tel: 415-864-7234
Dr. Misha Cohen, instructor
  Paths to Wholeness Professional Seminars are conducted by Misha Cohen, O.M.D., for Chinese medicine practitioners. The seminars include:

1. Quan Yin Professional HIV Certification—This is a postgraduate professional training program for acupuncturists, Chinese medicine practitioners, and M.D.s trained in traditional Chinese medicine.
2. Advanced HIV training seminars on digestive disorders, respiratory disorders, dermatological disorders, women's disorders.

Where to Study Chinese Medicine

Accreditation Commission for Acupuncture and Oriental Medicine (ACAOM)
1010 Wayne Avenue, Suite 1270
Silver Spring, MD 20910
Tel: 301-608-9680

ACAOM is the main accrediting body for Chinese medicine schools in the United States. You will find a full list of schools in *The Chinese Way to Healing: Many Paths to Wholeness,* by Misha Cohen (Perigee, 1996), or by contacting ACAOM.

Where to Get Chinese Herbs

No one should use Chinese herbs without the recommendation and supervision of a trained Chinese herbalist. For the general public there are a limited number of herbs that may be ordered over the counter without a prescription. The following companies or centers provide quality products to practitioners and sometimes to consumers.

For a more complete listing of suppliers of Chinese and Western herbs, contact the American Herbal Products Association, P.O. Box 2410, Austin, TX 78768, tel: 512-320-8555.

Brion Herb Corporation
9200 Jeronimo Road
Irvine, CA 92618
Tel: 800-333-4372

Brion, one of the oldest herbal companies in the United States, provides high-quality Sun Ten concentrated individual herbs and formulas. Practitioners may order special individualized formulations from Brion.

Health Concerns (for individuals and practitioners)
8001 Capwell Drive
Oakland, CA 94621
Tel: 800-233-9355
Fax: 510-639-9140
Andrew Gaeddert, president, herbalist

Health Concerns manufactures a line of general formulas for the public and distributes other products such as echinacea, tiger balm, etc. The company also manufactures a line of high-quality Chinese herbal formulas, including Enhance and other products designed by the author. Health Concerns maintains an herbal helpline for licensed practitioners. For the name of a licensed practitioner who uses this company's herbs, write or fax Health Concerns. Referrals are not given over the phone.

Kenshin Trading
1815 W. 213 Street, Suite 180
Torrance, CA 90501
   This company is a source for reishi mushrooms.

Mayway: China Native Herbs and Produce
1338 Mandela Parkway
Oakland, CA 94607
Tel: 510-208-3113
   Mayway is one of the largest and most reputable suppliers of Chinese herbal medicines in the United States.

Quan Yin Healing Arts Center
See page 208 for contact information.
   People with a written prescription from their licensed practitioner may buy herbs from Quan Yin in person or by mail. Those without a prescription must have a consultation before receiving herbs.

Where to Get Nutritional Supplements

The following four companies are mentioned because they supply supplements to Chicken Soup Chinese Medicine and Quan Yin. They may not sell to the general public but will recommend a practitioner in your area who carries these products. Many of the products are superior in quality and comparable or lower in price than supplements available in health food and vitamin stores.

Karuna: Responsible Nutrition
42 Digital Drive, Suite 7
Novato, CA 94949
Tel: 800-826-7225
   Karuna carries a wide variety of supplements and herbs for practitioner distribution only. I use this brand in my clinic for all the basic nutritional supplementation. I also use their Phytogest, a natural progesterone cream.

Natren, Inc.
3105 Willow Lane
Westlake Village, CA 91361
Tel: 800-992-3323
   A good source for acidophilus and pro-biotic products.

Transitions for Health
621 S.W. Alder, Suite 900
Portland, OR 97205
Tel: 800-888-6814
   A good source for progesterone products. There are many forms of natural pro-

gesterone on the market; we have used this company's Pro-gest Cream with good results.

Wholesale Nutrition
Box 3345
Saratoga, CA 95070
Tel: 800-325-2664
A good source for vitamin C (C-salts) in ascorbate form.

Professional Products for Practitioner Use

bio/chem Research
865 Parallel Drive
Lakeport, CA 95453
Tel: 707-263-1475
Fax: 707-263-7844
Richard Perry, president
Is the exclusive manufacturer of Citricidal grapefruit-seed extract, which is used for maintaining a healthy gastrointestinal tract. It is available in concentrated liquid, capsules, or tablets.

CompliMed Homeopathics, Inc.
1441 W. Smith Road
Ferndale, WA 98248
Tel: 360-384-5656; 800-232-4005
Fax: 360-384-1140
Jim Coyne, president
Technical support for practitioners: Mary Beth Watkins, director of research and development
Provides an extensive line of homeopathic combination remedies available in liquids, tablets, and creams.

McZand Herbal, Inc.
1722 14th Street, Suite 235
Boulder, CO 80302
Tel: 303-786-8558; 800-800-0405
Fax: 303-786-9435
Michael McGuffin, president
Its Chinese Classics is a full line of traditional Chinese formulas and individual herbs. Offered exclusively for the health care practitioner. They also provide custom dual extraction and blending of individual formulas.

NF Formulas, Inc.
9775 S.W. Commerce Circle, C-5
Wilsonville, OR 97070
Tel: 503-682-9755; 800-547-4891
Fax: 503-682-9529
Has nutritional supplements formulated by naturopathic physicians.

Spring Wind Herbs
2325 Fourth Street, #6
Berkeley, CA 94710
Tel: 510-849-1820; 800-588-4883 (orders)
Andrew Ellis, herbalist, owner

Spring Wind specializes in external topical formulas designed by Andrew Ellis, an accomplished herbalist and teacher. Spring Wind also supplies herbal concentrates and bulk herbs to practitioners. The quality of herbs is excellent. Practitioners may order individual herbal prescriptions from Spring Wind.

Women's Group Formulas, a division of Transitions for Health, Inc.
621 S.W. Alder, Suite 900
Portland, OR 97205
Tel: 503-226-1010; 800-861-5009
Fax: 800-861-8155; 503-226-6455
Sharon McFarland, CEO, owner
Technical support for practitioners, Debbie Moskowitz

Offers Pro-Gest Wild Yam Cream and other products for pre- and post-menopausal symptoms. The full line includes cream and oral drops, a phytoestrogen cream, and natural vaginal lubricant.

Appendix 5:

Publications

Publishers

Write or call any of these publishers for a list of available Chinese medicine titles.

Blue Poppy Press
1775 Linden Avenue
Boulder, CO 80304
Tel: 800-487-9296

Blue Poppy Press and its founder, Bob Flaws, are well known in the world of Chinese medicine. The press sells books for practitioners and the general public on a wide range of Chinese medicine topics.

China Books and Periodicals
2929 24th Street
San Francisco, CA 94110
Tel: 415-282-2994

Eastland Press
1260 Activity Drive, Suite A
Vista, CA 92083
Tel: 760-598-9695; 800-453-3278 (orders)
Fax: 800-241-3329 (orders)

Eastwind Books
1435 Stockton Street
San Francisco, CA 94133
Tel: 415-772-5899

This independent bookstore stocks the nation's most comprehensive selection of both Chinese- and English-language books on traditional Chinese medicine and nutrition, t'ai chi, Qi Gong, Chinese divination arts, Feng Shui, and Chinese philosophy.

Pacific View Press
P.O. Box 2657
Berkeley, CA 94702
Tel: 510-849-4213
Fax: 510-843-5835

Paradigm
P.O. Box 16982
San Diego, CA 92116
This company publishes only Chinese medicine books.

Pearson Professional Limited, Medical Division (U.S.A.)
650 Avenue of the Americas
New York, NY 10011
Tel: 212-727-7790
Attn: Churchill Livingstone

Redwing Book Company
44 Linden Street
Brookline, MA 04126
Tel: 800-873-3946 (orders)

Selected Books, Publications, and Web Sites

Acupuncture.com
Web address: www.acupuncture.com
Complete listing of acupuncturists across the country. Also has 500 Web pages covering all aspects of Chinese medicine for practitioners and consumers. Many links to other Chinese and alternative medicine Web sites. Also features exerpts from *The Chinese Way to Healing: Many Paths to Wholeness* and from this book.

AIDS, Immunity, and Chinese Medicine
Proceedings of the Ninth Annual Symposium of the Oriental Healing Arts Institute, held October 23, 1988 (published in 1989). Available from OHAI, 1945 Palo Verde Avenue, Suite 208, Long Beach, CA 90815.

AIDS Treatment News
P.O. Box 411256
San Francisco, CA 94141
Tel: 800-873-2812, 415-861-2432
Fax: 415-255-4659
Web address: www.aidsnews.org
John S. James, publisher, editor
Up-to-date information on treatment and clinical trials.

American Journal of Acupuncture
1840 41st Avenue, #102
P.O. Box 610
Capitola, CA 95010
Tel/fax: 408-475-1700

BETA Bulletin of Experimental Treatments for AIDS
P.O. Box 426182
San Francisco, CA 94142
Tel: 800-959-1059

Regular interactive phone conferences where you can call in and listen to experts discuss treatment issues. A project of the San Francisco AIDS Foundation.

Between Heaven and Earth: A Guide to Chinese Medicine (Ballantine Books, 1991).
By Harriet Beinfield, L.Ac., and Efrem Korngold, O.M.D., L.Ac.
Very popular introduction to Chinese medicine and the Five Phases types.

Centers for Disease Control
AIDS Web site with extensive information on all aspects of treatment; for publications call 800-458-5231 or visit their Web site: www.cdcnac.org.

Chinese Herbal Medicine, Formulas and Strategies (Eastland Press, 1990)
Compiled and translated by Dan Bensky and Randall Barolet.

Chinese Materia Medica (Eastland Press, 1986)
Compiled and translated by Dan Bensky and Andrew Gamble, with Ted Kaptchuk.

Cultivating Female Sexual Energy: Healing Love Through the Tao (Healing Tao Books, 1986)
By Mantak Chia and Maneewan Chia.

Guides for Living
Sue Pattyn
Tel: 303-702-1254
Fax: 303-702-1258
E-mail: pattyn@farragut.com
A listing of over 29,000 HIV/AIDS resources.

Gynecological Care Manual for HIV-Positive Women
By Risa Denenberg, F.N.P.
Essential Medical Information Systems, Inc.
Tel: 800-225-0694

Holistic Resource List for Treatment and Information about HIV/AIDS
Compiled by River Huston, 1997; distributed by the Women's Wellness Fund.
Women's Wellness Center
18 North Main Street
New Hope, PA 18938
For alternative and conventional therapies, lists of contact information such as newsletters, journals, fact sheets, organizations, Internet sites, practitioners, and information on women and children with HIV.

Immune Power: A Comprehensive Treatment for HIV (St. Martin's Press, 1993)
By John Kaiser, M.D.

Institute for Traditional Medicine
Web address: www.europa.com/itm
Subhuti Dharmananda, director

This site includes resources for practitioners, a listing of clinics for treatment of HIV infection, and information on herbal medicine.

Journal of the American College of Traditional Chinese Medicine
455 Arkansas Street
San Francisco, CA 94107
Tel: 415-282-7600
Although this journal is no longer being published, back issues and complete sets are still available from the college. They contain some excellent articles.

Journal of Chinese Medicine
c/o Eastland Press
1260 Activity Drive, Suite #A
Vista, CA 92083
Tel: 800-453-3278

Journal of the National Academy of Acupuncture and Oriental Medicine
28 Wildey Street
Tarrytown, NY 10591-3104
Tel: 800-257-6876

Nutrition and HIV: A New Model for Treatment, **second edition (Jossey-Bass, 1998)**
By Mary Romeyn, M.D.
This book, much updated from the very useful first edition, provides simple-to-follow dietary programs and nutritional supplement routines.

Nutrition for Life
Tufts University School of Medicine
136 Harrison Avenue
Boston, MA 0211
Tel: 617-636-0921
Fax: 617-636-5810
Free quarterly newsletter about nutrition and HIV infection.

Passion Play: Ancient Secrets to a Lifetime of Health and Happiness through Sensational Sex **(Riverhead Books, 1997)**
By Felice Dunas, Ph.D., with Philip Goldberg

The Positive Life: Portraits of Women Living with HIV **(Running Press, 1997)**
By River Huston; photographs by Mary Berridge

Positively Well: AIDS as a Chronic, Manageable, Survivable Disease **(Irvington Publishers, 1998)**
By Lark Lands, Ph.D.
Tel order line: 800-542-8102 (9 A.M.–5 P.M., EST)

POZ
349 W. 12th Street
New York, NY 10014
Tel: 212-242-1900
Monthly magazine for HIV-positive people featuring many articles on treatment, including on alternative therapies and Chinese medicine.

The Practice of Chinese Medicine: The Treatment of Disease with Acupuncture and Chinese Herbs **(Churchill Livingstone, 1994)**
By Giovanni Maciocia.
A textbook for serious students of Chinese medicine.

Psychoimmunity and the Healing Process: A Holistic Approach to Immunity and AIDS **(Celestial Arts, 1989)**
By Jason Serinus.
The book includes information on Chinese medicine and has input by Dr. Cohen.

The Web That Has No Weaver **(Congdon and Weed, 1983)**
By Ted Kaptchuk, O.M.D.
The first widely popular book on Chinese medicine theory published in the United States. It is used as a textbook in Chinese medicine classes worldwide.

Yin Yang Butterfly: Ancient Chinese Secrets for Western Lovers
(Tarcher/Putnam, 1994)
By Valentin Chu.

Appendix 6:

National Organizations

ACT UP: The AIDS Coalition to Unleash Power
HIV-positive people and their supporters who have influenced U.S. treatment policies through direct action. There is no centralized organization, so contact the branch in your area.

- **ACT UP Golden Gate, San Francisco**
  Tel: 415-252-9200

- **ACT UP New York**
  332 Bleeker Street, Suite G5
  New York, NY 10014
  Tel: 212-966-4873
  E-mail: actupny@panix.com

- **ACT UP Philadelphia**
  P.O. Box 15919
  Philadelphia, PA 19103
  Tel: 215-731-1844
  Fax: 215-731-1845
  E-mail: JDavids@critpath.org

AIDS and Chinese Medicine Institute (ACMI)
P.O. Box 14533
San Francisco, CA 94114-0533
Tel: 415-554-0154
Fax: 415-282-2935
E-mail: 73563.2131@compuserve.com
Howard Moffet, executive director

Center for Health Policy Development (CHPD)
6905 Alamo Downs Parkway
San Antonio, TX 78238
Tel: 800-847-7212
Fax: 210-520-9522
   CHPD addresses unmet and undermet health concerns of the Chicano population, including specific training in HIV/AIDS in Hispanic communities.

Critical Path AIDS Project

2062 Lombard Street
Philadelphia, PA 19146
Tel: 215-545-2212 (24-hour hotline)
Web address: www.critpath.org

The most comprehensive collection of articles and reprints on experimental treatments and alternative therapies. Web site has links to hundreds of other HIV/AIDS sites.

National AIDS Hotline

Tel: 800-342-AIDS, 800-344-SIDA *(en español),* 800-AIDS TTY (hearing impaired)

To find out about AIDS resources located in your area call the 24-hour hotline.

National Association of People with AIDS

1413 K Street NW, 7th Floor
Washington, DC 20005
Tel: 202-898-0414
Fax: 202-898-0435

Publishes newsletters and provides many membership benefits.

National Minority AIDS Council (NMAC)

1931 13th Street, NW
Washington, DC 20009-4432
Tel: 202-483-6622
Fax: 202-483-1135
E-mail: NMAC2@aol.com

NMAC has been a leader in advocacy and training for women and men of color. NMAC regularly sponsors national conferences and training sessions to develop organizational skills as well as create networks among community-based organizations that serve people of color with HIV.

National Pediatric and Family HIV Resource Center (NPHRC)

30 Bergen Street
Newark, NJ 07107
Tel: 800-362-0071
Fax: 201-972-0399
E-mail: NPHR@daiid.umdnj.edu

Project Inform

1965 Market Street, Suite 220
San Francisco, CA 94103
Tel: 415-558-8669; treatment hotline: 415-558-9051 or toll-free 800-822-7422
Fax: 415-558-8669
Web address: www.projinf.org

National nonprofit treatment information and advocacy organization that helps educate those with HIV infection on treatment and lifestyle strategies.

Project WISE

Part of Project Inform

Providing women with HIV with information.

Women Alive
1566 Burnside Avenue
Los Angeles, CA 90019
Tel: 213-965-1564
Fax: 213-965-9886

Women Alive publishes the *Women Alive Newsletter*, which includes listings of women's organizations and information for women not found elsewhere.

Women Organized to Respond to Life-Threatening Disease (WORLD)
P.O. Box 11535
Oakland CA 94611
Tel: 510-658-6930

Conducts HIV University to help women learn about HIV/AIDS and publishes a newsletter.

Women's AIDS Network (WAN)
3543 18th Street, Suite 11
San Francisco, CA 94110
Tel: 415-621-4160
Fax: 415-575-1181
Web address: www.womens-aids-network.com

Through a newsletter, educational forums, and a resource library, WAN advocates and provides development and improvement of public policies, education, and services for the diverse population of women infected and affected by HIV.

Appendix 7

The Buyers' Clubs

Buyers' clubs help people with AIDS and people at risk for AIDS obtain substances that for any reason are unavailable to them. This list was assembled by Critical Path AIDS Project, tel 215-545-2212 (24-hour hotline), 2062 Lombard Street, Philadelphia, PA 19146. All information was up-to-date as of January 1998.

AIDS Treatment Initiatives/Atlanta Buyers' Club
828 W. Peachtree Street, NW, Suite 210
Atlanta, GA 30308
Jamey Rousey, director

Being Alive Buyers' Club
111 E. Camelback Road
Phoenix, AZ 85012
Tel: 602-265-2437
Fax: 602-265-7201
Mark Hoffman, director
   A full-range club, but does not offer prescription medications.

Canadian Nutrition Club
275 Brockville Street
Smith Falls, Ontario, K7A 4Z6
Tel: 800-996-8466

Carl Vogel Foundation
1012 14 Street, NW, Suite 707
Washington, DC 20005
Tel: 202-638-0750
Fax: 202-638-0749
Ron Mealy, director
   Information on nutrition and alternative therapies, buyers' club. Write for some excellent reprints on the subject, such as "Therapeutic Basics for People Living with HIV," by Lark Lands, Ph.D.

CFIDS Buyers' Club
1187 Coast Village Road, #1-280
Santa Barbara, CA 93108
Tel: 800-366-6056

Direct AIDS Alternative Information Resources (DAAIR)
31 E. 30th Street, Suite 2A
New York, NY 10016
Tel: 212-725-6994
Fred Bingham, director
   New York City's alternative buyers' club. Ninety-five-page packet of information comes with membership; consultations available.

Healing Alternatives Foundation and Resource Library
1748 Market Street, #204
San Francisco, CA 94102
Tel: 415-626-4053 (to leave message)
E-mail: haf@sfbayguardian.com
   One of the oldest and most respected of the buyers' clubs. Maintains extensive public AIDS/HIV Treatment and Resource Library.

Health Link
3213 N. Ocean Boulevard, #6
Ft. Lauderdale, FL 33308
Tel: 954-565-8284
Fax: 954-565-8289
Marie Wansiki, director

Life Extension Buyers' Club
Life Extension Foundation
P.O. Box 229120
Hollywood, FL 33022
Also: 2490 Griffin Road
Ft. Lauderdale, FL 33312
Tel: 800-841-5433, 305-925-2500
Saul Kent, director
   They publish *Life Extension Report.*

LifeLink
750 Farroll Road
Grover Beach, CA 93433
Tel: 805-473-1389
David Blanco, director

PACT for Life Buyers' Club
P.O. Box 2488
Tucson, AZ 85702
Tel: 602-770-1710
Fax: 602-622-5822
Dan Nunez, director

PCA
1314 ¹/₂ E. Pine Street
Seattle, WA 98122
Tel: 206-526-2470
Greg Whiting, director

PWA Coop San Diego
4234 Oregon Street
San Diego, CA 92104

PWA Health Group
150 W. 26th Street, Suite 201
New York, NY 10001
Tel: 212-255-0520
Fax: 212-255-2080
Sally Cooper, director
   This large-volume buyers' club publishes *Notes from the Underground,* which features well-written and -researched articles on underground treatments.

Supplements Plus
2304 Bloor Street W
Toronto, Canada M6S 1P2
Fax: 416-766-2051
Stewart Brown, director
   Offers primarily vitamins and nutritional supplements.

Wholesale Health
909 N.E. 18th Street,
Ft. Lauderdale, FL 33305
Tel: 954-764-1587
Mel Smith, director

Appendix 8

Miscellaneous

Water Filters

Multi-Pure

Tel: 800-622-9206

I recommend that everyone filter their tap water. Multi-Pure is one source for reasonably priced high-quality water filters.

Stool Tests

Great Smokies Laboratories

63 Zillicoa Street
Asheville, NC 28801
Tel: 800-522-4762; 704-253-0621

This lab is one of very few in the United States that provides extremely accurate stool tests. Ask your doctor for more information.

Qi Gong for Health (San Francisco)

Tel: 415-661-2080
Contact: George Wedemeyer

Offers classes and a videotape specifically for HIV-positive people.

Qi Gong Institute

561 Berkeley Avenue
Menlo Park, CA 94025
E-mail: qigonginstitute@nanospace.com
Web address: www.healthy.net/qigonginstitute
Kenneth Sancier, Ph.D., president

The Qi Gong Institute promotes medical Qi Gong via education, research, and clinical studies. Makes available information on Qi Gong and its integration with Western medicine.

Qi Gong and Tai Chi Chuan Videotapes

***Wong's Taiji and Qi Gong for Health,* by Larry Wong**
1775 21st Avenue
San Francisco, CA 94122
Tel: 415-753-0426

Interviews with Larry Wong formed the basis of the chapter on Qi Gong in *The Chinese Way to Healing: Many Paths to Wholeness* (Perigee, 1996), and this book.

Soy Foods

The Soy Foods Center
Lafayette, CA 94549
William Shurtleff, director

The world's leading center for information on soy foods.

Index

 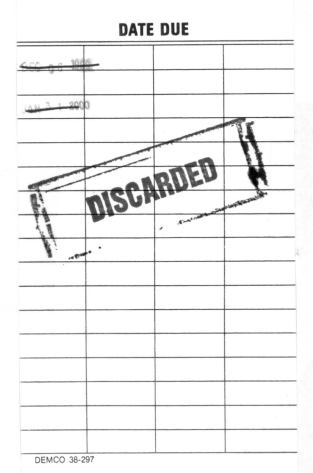